Noom Diet Cookbook for Beginners 2024

The Complete 100+ Healthy and Delicious Recipes To Improve Metabolism And Lose Weight

BONUS: Meal plan + Video course

Dr. Phyllis Olsen

Copyright © 2024 by Dr. Phyllis Olsen

All rights reserved. No part of this book may be reproduced or transmitted in any form or by any means, electronic or mechanical, including photocopying, recording, or by any information storage and retrieval system, without permission in writing from the copyright owner.

About the Author

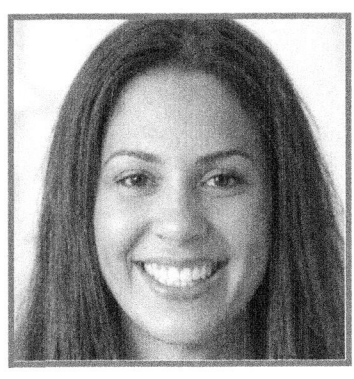

Reputable authority on culinary health, Dr. Phyllis Olsen specializes in developing delectable dishes that support long-term weight management. With a PhD in nutritional sciences, Dr. Olsen has devoted her professional life to leveraging people's love of cooking to help them reach their health objectives.

Dr. Olsen is a fervent supporter of healthy living, and her knowledge is evident in her specialty cookbooks, which are designed to make losing weight a tasty and joyful experience. Her creative approach to fusing delicious food with nutrition has won her recognition from the culinary and medical sectors.

Dr. Olsen offers readers more than just delicious recipes; with years of study and real-world experience, she has amassed a wealth of information that has helped her understand the science behind balanced eating. Her dedication to advocating for a comprehensive and enduring strategy for managing weight distinguishes her writing in the field of culinary literature.

In addition to being a skilled writer, Dr. Olsen uses online forums, seminars, and workshops to actively interact with her audience. She is committed to creating a community of people who are enthusiastic about health and offers constant support and direction.

Phyllis Olsen's publications attest to her conviction that leading a healthy lifestyle ought to be enjoyable and fulfilling. Through the pages of her motivational cookbooks, go on a journey with her to learn about the relationship between culinary creativity and wellbeing.

Connect with Dr. Olsen for the most recent information, recipes, and health advice.

Bonus

Day 1

Breakfast: Greek Yogurt Parfait
Lunch: Grilled Chicken Salad
Dinner: Baked Cod with Lemon and Herbs
Snack: Guacamole with Veggie Sticks

Day 2

Breakfast: Avocado Toast
Lunch: Quinoa and Black Bean Bowl
Dinner: Vegetarian Chili
Snack: Greek Yogurt and Berry Parfait

Day 3

Breakfast: Banana Nut Smoothie
Lunch: Turkey and Veggie Wrap
Dinner: Teriyaki Tofu Stir-Fry
Snack: Hummus and Veggie Platter

Day 4

Breakfast: Oatmeal with Berries
Lunch: Vegetable Stir-Fry
Dinner: Pesto Chicken and Veggie Skewers
Snack: Cottage Cheese and Pineapple Salsa

Day 5

Breakfast: Egg White Scramble
Lunch: Salmon and Asparagus
Dinner: Spaghetti Squash with Marinara
Snack: Baked Sweet Potato Fries

Day 6

Breakfast: Whole Grain Pancakes

Lunch: Caprese Salad
Dinner: Salmon and Quinoa Salad
Snack: Caprese Skewers

Day 7

Breakfast: Chia Seed Pudding
Lunch: Shrimp and Broccoli Stir-Fry
Dinner: Stuffed Bell Peppers with Turkey
Snack: Edamame with Sea Salt

Day 8

Breakfast: Smoothie Bowl
Lunch: Mediterranean Chickpea Salad
Dinner: Lemon Garlic Shrimp Pasta
Snack: Apple Slices with Almond Butter

Day 9

Breakfast: Quinoa Breakfast Bowl
Lunch: Veggie Wrap with Hummus
Dinner: Eggplant Parmesan
Snack: Kale Chips

Day 10

Breakfast: Vegetable Omelette
Lunch: Tuna Salad Lettuce Wraps
Dinner: Cauliflower Pizza Crust
Snack: Vegetable Spring Rolls

Day 11

Breakfast: Peanut Butter Banana Wrap
Lunch: Sweet Potato and Black Bean Bowl
Dinner: Turkey and Sweet Potato Skillet
Snack: Roasted Chickpeas

Day 12

Breakfast: Cottage Cheese with Pineapple
Lunch: Chicken Caesar Salad
Dinner: Sesame Ginger Salmon
Snack: Mixed Berry Smoothie Popsicles

Day 13

Breakfast: Whole Grain Waffles
Lunch: Quinoa Stuffed Peppers
Dinner: Chickpea and Spinach Curry
Snack: Trail Mix

Day 14

Breakfast: Breakfast Burrito
Lunch: Lentil Soup
Dinner: Mushroom and Spinach Stuffed Chicken
Snack: Stuffed Mini Bell Peppers

Day 15

Breakfast: Apple Cinnamon Overnight Oats
Lunch: Turkey and Quinoa Meatballs
Dinner: Quinoa and Vegetable Stir-Fry
Snack: Cucumber Slices with Tzatziki

Day 16

Breakfast: Sweet Potato Hash
Lunch: Veggie Wrap with Avocado
Dinner: Sweet Potato and Black Bean Enchiladas
Snack: Almond and Dark Chocolate Clusters

Day 17

Breakfast: Mango Coconut Smoothie
Lunch: Pesto Zoodles with Cherry Tomatoes
Dinner: Lemon Herb Grilled Shrimp
Snack: Roasted Red Pepper Hummus Wrap

Day 18

Breakfast: Blueberry Almond Muffins
Lunch: Chickpea and Spinach Salad
Dinner: Turkey and Veggie Skillet
Snack: Tomato Basil Bruschetta

Day 19

Breakfast: Egg and Veggie Muffins
Lunch: Cauliflower Fried Rice
Dinner: Zucchini Noodles with Pesto
Snack: Avocado and Tomato Salsa

Day 20

Breakfast: Peach Almond Smoothie
Lunch: Egg Salad Lettuce Wraps
Dinner: Baked Chicken with Rosemary and Lemon
Snack: Greek Yogurt Dipped Strawberries

Day 21

Breakfast: Spinach and Feta Breakfast Wrap
Lunch: Blackened Chicken Salad
Dinner: Vegetable and Quinoa Stuffed Portobello Mushrooms
Snack: Sliced Bell Peppers with Cottage Cheese

Day 22

Breakfast: Grilled Chicken Salad
Lunch: Quinoa and Black Bean Bowl
Dinner: Teriyaki Tofu Stir-Fry
Snack: Greek Yogurt and Berry Parfait

Day 23

Breakfast: Banana Nut Smoothie
Lunch: Turkey and Veggie Wrap

Dinner: Pesto Chicken and Veggie Skewers
Snack: Hummus and Veggie Platter

Day 24

Breakfast: Oatmeal with Berries
Lunch: Vegetable Stir-Fry
Dinner: Spaghetti Squash with Marinara
Snack: Baked Sweet Potato Fries

Day 25

Breakfast: Egg White Scramble
Lunch: Salmon and Asparagus
Dinner: Stuffed Bell Peppers with Turkey
Snack: Caprese Skewers

Day 26

Breakfast: Whole Grain Pancakes
Lunch: Caprese Salad
Dinner: Salmon and Quinoa Salad
Snack: Cottage Cheese and Pineapple Salsa

Day 27

Breakfast: Chia Seed Pudding
Lunch: Shrimp and Broccoli Stir-Fry
Dinner: Quinoa and Vegetable Stir-Fry
Snack: Edamame with Sea Salt

Your Video Course is here!!!

To get your video course, kindly insert the below link into your browser:

http://tinyurl.com/y75w7zve

Or scan the below QR code:

Table of content

Introduction..8
   Overview of the Noom Diet..8
   Benefits of Following the Noom Diet..9
   Getting Started with the Cookbook...9

Chapter 1: Understanding the Noom Diet...11
   Principles and Philosophy..11
   How the Noom Diet Improves Metabolism...11
   Role of Noom Color Codes..12

Chapter 2: Essential Tools and Ingredients..13
   Kitchen Tools for Noom Cooking..13
   Must-Have Ingredients in Your Pantry..13
   Shopping Tips for Noom Diet Followers...14

Chapter 3: Breakfast Recipes...15
   Greek Yogurt Parfait..15
   Avocado Toast...16
   Banana Nut Smoothie..17
   Oatmeal with Berries...18
   Egg White Scramble..19
   Whole Grain Pancakes..20
   Chia Seed Pudding..21
   Smoothie Bowl..22
   Quinoa Breakfast Bowl..23
   Vegetable Omelet..24
   Egg and Veggie Muffins...26
   Peach Almond Smoothie...27
   Spinach and Feta Breakfast Wrap..28

Chapter 4: Lunch Ideas..29
   Grilled Chicken Salad..29
   Quinoa and Black Bean Bowl..31
   Turkey and Veggie Wrap..32
   Vegetable Stir-Fry..34
   Salmon and Asparagus...35
   Caprese Salad...36
   Shrimp and Broccoli Stir-Fry..37
   Mediterranean Chickpea Salad..39
   Veggie Wrap with Hummus..40
   Tuna Salad Lettuce Wraps...41
   Sweet Potato and Black Bean Bowl...42
   Chicken Caesar Salad...43

Quinoa Stuffed Peppers 44
Lentil Soup 46
Turkey and Quinoa Meatballs 48
Veggie Wrap with Avocado 50
Pesto Zoodles with Cherry Tomatoes 51
Chickpea and Spinach Salad 53
Cauliflower Fried Rice 54
Egg Salad Lettuce Wraps 56
Blackened Chicken Salad 57

Chapter 5: Dinner Delights 58
Baked Cod with Lemon and Herbs 58
Vegetarian Chili 59
Teriyaki Tofu Stir-Fry 60
Pesto Chicken and Veggie Skewers 61
Spaghetti Squash with Marinara 62
Salmon and Quinoa Salad 63
Stuffed Bell Peppers with Turkey 64
Lemon Garlic Shrimp Pasta 65
Eggplant Parmesan 66
Cauliflower Pizza Crust 67
Turkey and Sweet Potato Skillet 68
Sesame Ginger Salmon 69
Chickpea and Spinach Curry 70
Mushroom and Spinach Stuffed Chicken 71
Quinoa and Vegetable Stir-Fry 72
Sweet Potato and Black Bean Enchiladas 73
Lemon Herb Grilled Shrimp 74
Turkey and Veggie Skillet 75
Zucchini Noodles with Pesto 76
Baked Chicken with Rosemary and Lemon 77
Vegetable and Quinoa Stuffed Portobello Mushrooms 78

Chapter 6: Snacks and Appetizers 79
Guacamole with Veggie Sticks 79
Greek Yogurt and Berry Parfait 80
Hummus and Veggie Platter 81
Cottage Cheese and Pineapple Salsa 82
Baked Sweet Potato Fries 83
Caprese Skewers 84
Edamame with Sea Salt 85
Apple Slices with Almond Butter 86
Kale Chips 87

Vegetable Spring Rolls..........88
Roasted Chickpeas..........89
Mixed Berry Smoothie Popsicles..........90
Trail Mix..........91
Stuffed Mini Bell Peppers..........92
Cucumber Slices with Tzatziki..........93
Almond and Dark Chocolate Clusters..........94
Roasted Red Pepper Hummus Wrap..........95
Tomato Basil Bruschetta..........96
Avocado and Tomato Salsa..........97
Greek Yogurt Dipped Strawberries..........98
Sliced Bell Peppers with Cottage Cheese..........99

Chapter 7: Desserts for the Noom Diet..........100
Mixed Berry Frozen Yogurt..........100
Dark Chocolate-Dipped Banana Slices..........101
Baked Apples with Cinnamon..........102
Chia Seed Pudding with Mango..........103
Frozen Grapes..........104
Coconut and Berry Parfait..........105
Pineapple Sorbet..........106
Yogurt and Berry Bark..........107
Mango and Mint Sorbet..........108
Almond and Date Energy Bites..........109
Watermelon Popsicles..........110
Berry Compote with Greek Yogurt..........111
Kiwi and Banana Ice Cream..........112
Chocolate Avocado Mousse..........113
Cinnamon Baked Pears..........114
Blueberry Coconut Chia Pudding..........115
Peach Frozen Yogurt Pops..........116
Vanilla Pomegranate Parfait..........117
Raspberry Almond Butter Bites..........118
Strawberry Shortcake..........119
Mango Coconut Chia Seed Popsicles..........120

Chapter 8: Meal Planning and Prepping..........121
Weekly Meal Plans..........121
Batch Cooking for Noom Success..........121
Tips for Efficient Meal Preparation..........122

Chapter 9: Staying Motivated on the Noom Diet..........123

Chapter 10: Frequently Asked Questions..........125
Common Noom Diet Queries..........125

Troubleshooting Guide...125
Additional Resources for Readers..126
Conclusion..**128**
Summary of Noom Diet Advantages:...128
Encouragement for Continued Success:..128

Introduction

Setting out on a quest for a healthy way of life may be intimidating as well as thrilling. With a wealth of delicious dishes and an in-depth explanation of the Noom Diet, the Noom Diet Cookbook for Beginners 2024 is here to help you navigate this journey. This introduction lays the groundwork for a meal that transcends beyond appearances and has a profound gastronomic impact.

Overview of the Noom Diet

The Noom Diet is a colorful and simple method to make thoughtful food choices; it's not your average restricted diet. It is essentially a color-coded system that divides foods into categories that are green, yellow, and red. The Noom Diet is based on an understanding of these colors.

Similar to fruits and vegetables, green meals are rich in nutrients and low in calories. They are the unsung heroes of your diet, providing you with necessary fiber, vitamins, and minerals without packing on the pounds. We'll discuss the advantages of eating a greater variety of green vegetables and how they improve your health in general.

Foods that are yellow have a modest calorie density. Lean proteins, whole grains, and certain dairy products are a few of them. Learn how eating foods that are yellow may provide you a balanced energy supply that will keep you full and energized all day.

Red foods, which include processed snacks, candies, and fatty meat cuts, have a greater calorie density. Red foods aren't forbidden, but we'll talk about how to eat them in moderation and find a balance that supports your health objectives.

It is not necessary to commit a list of dos and don'ts to memory in order to comprehend the Noom Diet; rather, one must adopt a sustainable and adaptable eating style. This chapter explores the theory of the Noom Diet, stressing the value of balance, diversity, and moderation.

Benefits of Following the Noom Diet

The Noom Diet: Why select it? The advantages go much beyond the assurance of losing weight. This chapter delves into the ways in which the Noom Diet may improve your general health and wellbeing.

Enhanced metabolism is a primary benefit of the Noom Diet. Learn how eating nutrient-dense meals and adopting wise eating practices may boost your metabolism and result in greater energy and effective burning of calories.

The secret to sustainable weight reduction is to develop long-lasting behaviors rather than merely dropping pounds. We'll talk about how the Noom Diet emphasizes small, doable adjustments that lead to long-term success. This is a change in lifestyle, not a band-aid solution.

We'll also look at how the Noom Diet supports mental health. The Noom method tackles the psychological components of feeding by promoting mindful eating and cultivating a good connection with food. This technique also lowers stress levels and encourages healthy thinking.

Getting Started with the Cookbook

It's critical to create the conditions for success before you begin working with the recipes. You will leave this chapter with the information and resources necessary to confidently follow the Noom Diet.

Find out which kitchen essentials are needed to make cooking with Noom a breeze. We'll walk you through the process of assembling a kitchen toolkit that guarantees precise and effective meal preparation, from measuring cups to kitchen scales.

Check out the essential components for your Nook pantry next. We'll break down the essential elements of a well-stocked kitchen, so you can easily prepare delicious and nourishing meals without having to worry about rushing to the store at the last minute.

Lastly, get insightful advice for shrewd supermarket buying. We'll provide advice on how to make decisions that are in line with the Noom Diet's tenets, from reading food labels to choosing the freshest fruit.

Chapter 1: Understanding the Noom Diet

Principles and Philosophy

The Noom diet is a comprehensive approach to health that integrates behavioral modification, nutrition science, and psychology. It's not only about losing weight. Noom is fundamentally based on the idea of making conscious, sustainable decisions. It helps users recognize triggers, better understand their connection with food, and form healthy behaviors.

Noom's ideology is centered on the concept of "cognitive restructuring." This entails changing people's perspectives on nutrition, physical activity, and general wellbeing. Noom offers a flexible framework that fits different lifestyles in place of rigid restrictions. It seeks to establish long-lasting habits that result in a healthy life by concentrating on the psychological side of eating.

How the Noom Diet Improves Metabolism

The Noom diet incorporates techniques to increase metabolic efficiency since it understands that metabolism plays a critical role in weight control. The focus on nutrient-dense meals that efficiently power the body is one important component. Noom promotes consuming proteins, carbs, and fats in a balanced manner, giving the body the building blocks it needs for a healthy metabolism.

Furthermore, Noom's strategy includes frequent physical exercise as a key component. Exercise helps people lose weight sustainably by increasing metabolic rate in addition to burning calories. Everyone may use Noom's individualized training regimens since they are designed to accommodate different fitness levels.

The Noom diet's emphasis on slow, consistent weight reduction has been shown in recent research to have a good effect on metabolism. Fast weight reduction often results in loss of muscle and a drop in metabolic rate; Noom's method strives for a more gradual and metabolism-friendly loss of weight.

Role of Noom Color Codes

More than simply a visual aid, Noom's distinctive color-coded system is an intelligent approach to classify and comprehend the nutritional content of various meals. Green, yellow, and red are the colors that assist people in making well-informed food selections.

Green foods are nutrient-dense, low-calorie meals that often include fruits and vegetables. Noom promotes consuming a lot of green vegetables since they are high in fiber, vitamins, and minerals and low in calories.

Yellow Foods: Whole grains, lean meats, and certain dairy products fall under this group. Foods that are yellow have a decent nutritional balance and a modest calorie density.

Red foods: They have more calories and often include processed and sugary foods. While Noom doesn't categorize red foods as "bad," it does advise eating them in moderation and with awareness.

Meal planning becomes an easy and informative procedure with Noom thanks to these color codes. Users progressively learn how to prepare colorful, well-balanced meals that help them reach their weight and health objectives.

Chapter 2: Essential Tools and Ingredients

Kitchen Tools for Noom Cooking

Cooking may be easy and pleasant if you have the proper equipment in your kitchen. There are just a few necessities to help you on your path to healthy eating—no costly devices required.

1. **Food Scale**: Accuracy in measuring ingredients is ensured by a sturdy food scale, which is important for portion management.

2. **Measuring Cups and Spoons**: In line with Noom's focus on mindful eating, these instruments aid in portion control and recipe uniformity.

3. **Steamer Basket**: Perfect for cooking veggies that are high in nutrients without sacrificing vital vitamins and minerals.

4. **Non-Stick Cookware**: Using non-stick cookware reduces the need for unnecessary cooking oils and encourages healthy food preparation.

5. **Blender or food processor**: Needed to make healthy soups, sauces, and smoothies using entire, fresh ingredients.

Must-Have Ingredients in Your Pantry

Having Noom-friendly products in your cupboard can help you succeed. Use this list as a help when you go food shopping:

1. **Whole Grains**: Complex carbs and fiber from whole wheat pasta, quinoa, brown rice, and oats help you feel satiated for longer.

2. **Lean Proteins**: Foods high in protein but low in saturated fats include lentils, fish, poultry, and tofu.

3. Nuts, seeds, avocados, and olive oil are good sources of monounsaturated fats that promote general health.

4. **Colorful Vegetables**: Incorporate a range of fresh and frozen vegetables into your meals to enhance taste, texture, and nutritional value.

5. **Fresh Fruits**: Not only do these naturally sweet delights fulfill your sweet need, but they also provide vitamins and antioxidants.

6. **Herbs and Spices**: Use seasonings, herbs, and spices to add flavor to your food without adding extra calories.

Shopping Tips for Noom Diet Followers

Making thoughtful plans and strategic decisions is necessary while navigating the grocery shop with the Noom mindset:

1. **Adhere to the Perimeter**: Fresh vegetables, lean meats, and dairy products—essential elements of the Noom diet—are usually found on the outer aisles.

2. Read ingredient labels carefully. Pay attention to added sugars, saturated fats, and highly processed foods. Choose items made mostly of whole foods.

3. **Make a list and plan your meals**: Being organized is essential. To prevent impulsive purchases, plan your meals for the next week, make a shopping list, and follow it.

4. **Visit the Farmers' Market**: Noom's focus on complete, less processed cuisine often pairs nicely with fresh, locally grown vegetables.

5. **Purchasing basics in quantity**: To guarantee you always have Noom-approved basics on hand and to save money, buy non-perishable goods in quantity.

Chapter 3: Breakfast Recipes

Greek Yogurt Parfait

Servings: 1
Cooking Time: 0 minutes
Prep Time: 5 minutes
Total Time: 5 minutes

Ingredients

1 cup Greek yogurt
1/2 cup granola
1/4 cup fresh berries
1 tablespoon honey

Instructions

1. Arrange Greek yogurt layers in a glass or dish.
2. Top with granola.
3. Top the granola with some fresh berries.
4. For sweetness, drizzle with honey.
5. Continue layering as needed.
6. Savor your mouth watering parfait of Greek yogurt!

Nutritional Information

Calories: 300
Fat: 10g
Protein: 20g
Carbohydrates: 35g
Cholesterol: 10mg

Avocado Toast

Servings: 1
Cooking Time: 5 minutes
Prep Time: 5 minutes
Total Time: 10 minutes

Ingredients

1 slice whole-grain bread
1 ripe avocado
Salt and pepper to taste
Optional toppings: poached egg, cherry tomatoes, red pepper flakes

Instructions

1. Make your own toast with whole-grain bread.
2. Top the toasted bread with the mashed avocado.
3. Season with pepper and salt to taste.
4. If desired, add the optional toppings.
5. Avocado Toast is prepared for consumption!

Nutritional Information

Calories: 250
Fat: 15g
Protein: 6g
Carbohydrates: 25g
Cholesterol: 0mg

Banana Nut Smoothie

Servings: 1
Cooking Time: 0 minutes
Prep Time: 5 minutes
Total Time: 5 minutes

Ingredients

1 ripe banana
1/4 cup chopped nuts (almonds or walnuts)
1 cup milk (dairy or plant-based)
1 tablespoon honey
Ice cubes (optional)

Instructions

1. Place ripe banana, chopped almonds, milk, and honey in a blender.
2. Process until smooth.
3. Blend once more after adding ice cubes, if desired.
4. Fill a glass with the banana nut smoothie and enjoy!

Nutritional Information

Calories: 350
Fat: 18g
Protein: 8g
Carbohydrates: 45g
Cholesterol: 5mg

Oatmeal with Berries

Servings: 2
Cooking Time: 10 minutes
Prep Time: 2 minutes
Total Time: 12 minutes

Ingredients

1 cup rolled oats
2 cups milk (dairy or plant-based)
1/2 cup mixed berries (strawberries, blueberries, raspberries)
2 tablespoons maple syrup
Optional toppings: sliced bananas, chopped nuts

Instructions

1. Place the milk and rolled oats in a saucepan.
2. Cook the oats over medium heat, stirring from time to time, until the required consistency is reached.
3. Sort the oats into dishes.
4. Drizzle with maple syrup and garnish with a mixture of berries.
5. If desired, add the optional toppings.
6. It's time to serve your oatmeal with berries!

Nutritional Information

Calories: 300
Fat: 8g
Protein: 10g
Carbohydrates: 45g
Cholesterol: 5mg

Egg White Scramble

Servings: 2
Cooking Time: 8 minutes
Prep Time: 5 minutes
Total Time: 13 minutes

Ingredients

4 egg whites
1 cup spinach, chopped
1/2 cup cherry tomatoes, halved
1/4 cup feta cheese, crumbled
Salt and pepper to taste
1 tablespoon olive oil

Instructions

1. Beat the egg whites until foamy in a bowl.
2. In a pan over medium heat, warm the olive oil.
3. Add the chopped spinach and cherry tomato halves, and cook until the spinach wilts.
4. Add the whisked egg whites and give it a little swirl.
5. Cook the eggs until they are firm but not dry.
6. Top the scramble with crumbled feta cheese.
7. To taste, add salt and pepper for seasoning.
8. Present your mouth watering Egg White Scramble!

Nutritional Information

Calories: 180
Fat: 10g
Protein: 20g
Carbohydrates: 5g
Cholesterol: 5mg

Whole Grain Pancakes

Servings: 4
Cooking Time: 15 minutes
Prep Time: 10 minutes
Total Time: 25 minutes

Ingredients

1 cup whole wheat flour
1 tablespoon baking powder
1 tablespoon honey
1 cup milk (dairy or plant-based)
1 egg
2 tablespoons melted butter or oil
1 teaspoon vanilla extract

Instructions

1. Combine the baking powder and whole wheat flour in a bowl.
2. Combine honey, milk, egg, melted oil or butter, and vanilla extract in another dish.
3. Add the wet mixture to the dry mixture and whisk just until blended.
4. Turn up the heat to medium on a skillet or griddle.
5. For each pancake, pour 1/4 cup of batter onto the griddle.
6. Cook until surface bubbles appear, then turn and continue cooking until golden brown.
7. Top your whole grain pancakes with the toppings of your choice!

Nutritional Information

Calories: 150 (per pancake)
Fat: 6g
Protein: 4g
Carbohydrates: 20g
Cholesterol: 30mg

Chia Seed Pudding

Servings: 2
Prep Time: 5 minutes (plus chilling time)
Total Time: 4 hours (chilling time)

Ingredients

1/4 cup chia seeds
1 cup milk (dairy or plant-based)
1 tablespoon honey
1/2 teaspoon vanilla extract
Fresh fruit for topping

Instructions

1. Combine the chia seeds, milk, honey, and vanilla essence in a dish.
2. With periodic stirring, cover and chill for at least 4 hours or overnight.
3. Spoon into serving glasses when it has thickened.
4. Add your preferred fresh fruit on top.
5. You may now savor your Chia Seed Pudding!

Nutritional Information

Calories: 180 (per serving)
Fat: 8g
Protein: 5g
Carbohydrates: 25g
Cholesterol: 0mg

Smoothie Bowl

Servings: 1
Prep Time: 10 minutes
Total Time: 10 minutes

Ingredients

1 frozen banana
1/2 cup frozen berries (mixed or your choice)
1/2 cup yogurt (dairy or plant-based)
1 tablespoon almond butter
Toppings: granola, sliced banana, chia seeds, honey

Instructions

1. Place frozen banana, frozen berries, yogurt, and almond butter in a blender; process until smooth.
2. Transfer the blended drink to a basin.
3. Add granola, banana slices, chia seeds, and honey drizzle over top.
4. You may now enjoy your colorful smoothie bowl!

Nutritional Information

Calories: 350
Fat: 12g
Protein: 10g
Carbohydrates: 55g
Cholesterol: 5mg

Quinoa Breakfast Bowl

Servings: 2
Cooking Time: 15 minutes
Prep Time: 10 minutes
Total Time: 25 minutes

Ingredients

1 cup cooked quinoa
1/2 cup Greek yogurt
1/4 cup mixed nuts and seeds (almonds, pumpkin seeds)
1/2 cup fresh fruit (berries, sliced banana)
1 tablespoon honey

Instructions

1. Arrange the cooked quinoa in a bowl.
2. Add Greek yogurt on top.
3. Garnish the yogurt with a mixture of nuts and seeds.
4. Garnish with fresh fruit.
5. Add a honey drizzle for sweetness.
6. You are now prepared to serve your wholesome Quinoa Breakfast Bowl!

Nutritional Information

Calories: 300 (per serving)
Fat: 12g
Protein: 15g
Carbohydrates: 35g
Cholesterol: 5mg

Vegetable Omelet

Servings: 1
Cooking Time: 10 minutes
Prep Time: 5 minutes
Total Time: 15 minutes

Ingredients

3 large eggs
1/2 bell pepper, diced
1/4 cup diced onion
1/2 cup cherry tomatoes, halved
1/4 cup shredded cheese (cheddar or your choice)
Salt and pepper to taste
1 tablespoon olive oil

Instructions

1. Grease a muffin tray with paper liners and preheat the oven to 350°F (175°C).
2. Combine the almond flour, coconut flour, baking soda, baking powder, and salt in a bowl.
3. Beat the eggs in another dish and stir in the almond milk, melted coconut oil, vanilla extract, honey or maple syrup.
4. Gently stir the wet mixture into the dry mixture until it barely comes together.
5. Add the blueberries and fold.
6. Fill muffin tins with batter, and bake for 18 to 20 minutes, or until a toothpick inserted into the center comes out clean.
7. Before serving, let the muffins cool.

Nutritional Information

Calories: 200 (per muffin)
Fat: 15g
Protein: 5g
Carbohydrates: 15g
Cholesterol: 40mg

Egg and Veggie Muffins

Servings: 6
Cooking Time: 20 minutes
Prep Time: 10 minutes
Total Time: 30 minutes

Ingredients

6 large eggs
1/2 cup diced bell peppers
1/2 cup diced tomatoes
1/4 cup diced onions
1/4 cup chopped spinach
Salt and pepper to taste
1/2 cup shredded cheese (optional)

Instructions

1. Oil a muffin tray and preheat the oven to 375°F (190°C).
2. Whisk the eggs in a bowl and add pepper and salt to taste.
3. Add chopped spinach, tomatoes, onions, and diced bell peppers.
4. Using a measuring cup, fill each muffin cup approximately two thirds of the way up.
5. You may choose to top with shredded cheese.
6. Bake the eggs for 15 to 18 minutes, or until they set.
7. Let the muffins cool somewhat before taking them out of the muffin pan.

Nutritional Information

Calories: 120 (per muffin)
Fat: 8g
Protein: 8g
Carbohydrates: 4g
Cholesterol: 185mg

Peach Almond Smoothie

Servings: 1
Prep Time: 5 minutes
Total Time: 5 minutes

Ingredients

1 cup fresh or frozen peaches
1/2 cup almond milk
1/2 cup Greek yogurt
1 tablespoon almond butter
1 tablespoon honey
Ice cubes (optional)

Instructions

1. Put the peaches, Greek yogurt, almond butter, honey, and almond milk into a blender.
2. Process until smooth.
3. Blend once more after adding ice cubes, if desired.
4. Transfer into a glass, then enjoy your cool peach almond smoothie

Nutritional Information

Calories: 300
Fat: 15g
Protein: 10g
Carbohydrates: 35g
Cholesterol: 10mg

Spinach and Feta Breakfast Wrap

Servings: 1
Cooking Time: 5 minutes
Prep Time: 5 minutes
Total Time: 10 minutes

Ingredients

1 large whole wheat tortilla
2 large eggs, scrambled
Handful of fresh spinach
2 tablespoons crumbled feta cheese
Salt and pepper to taste
1 teaspoon olive oil

Instructions

1. Heat the olive oil in a skillet over medium heat.
2. Cook the fresh spinach until it wilts.
3. Transfer the scrambled eggs to the skillet and allow them to set.
4. Add pepper and salt for seasoning.
5. Top the whole wheat tortilla with the scrambled eggs and spinach.
6. Top with feta cheese crumbles.
7. Create a wrap by rolling up the tortilla.
8. You may now savor your delicious breakfast wrap with spinach and feta!

Nutritional Information

Calories: 400
Fat: 20g
Protein: 20g
Carbohydrates: 35g
Cholesterol: 370mg

Chapter 4: Lunch Ideas

Grilled Chicken Salad

Servings: 4
Cooking Time: 15 minutes
Prep Time: 20 minutes
Total Time: 35 minutes

Ingredients

2 boneless, skinless chicken breasts
8 cups mixed salad greens
1 cup cherry tomatoes, halved
1 cucumber, sliced
1/2 red onion, thinly sliced
1/4 cup feta cheese, crumbled
1/4 cup balsamic vinaigrette dressing

Instructions

1. Turn the heat up to medium-high on the grill.
2. Sprinkle salt and pepper on the chicken breasts.
3. Cook the chicken thoroughly, about 6 to 8 minutes on each side on the grill.
4. Give the chicken five minutes to rest before slicing.
5. Combine salad greens, cucumber, red onion, cherry tomatoes, and feta cheese in a big bowl.
6. Place sliced grilled chicken over the salad.
7. Cover the salad with a balsamic vinaigrette dressing.
8. Gently toss to mix and proceed to serve.

Nutritional Information(per serving)

Calories: 320
Fat: 12g
Protein: 30g
Carbohydrates: 20g
Fiber: 4g

Cholesterol: 80mg

Quinoa and Black Bean Bowl

Servings: 2
Cooking Time: 20 minutes
Prep Time: 10 minutes
Total Time: 30 minutes

Ingredients

1 cup quinoa, rinsed
2 cups water or vegetable broth
One can (15 oz) of black beans, washed and drained
1 cup corn kernels
1 avocado, diced
1/4 cup cilantro, chopped
1 lime, juiced
Salt and pepper to taste

Instructions

1. Put the quinoa and water (or veggie broth) in a medium pot. After bringing to a boil, lower the heat, cover, and simmer the quinoa for 15 minutes, or until it is tender.
2. Combine cooked quinoa, black beans, corn, avocado, and cilantro in a big bowl.
3. Sprinkle the mixture with lime juice and give it a little shake.
4. Season with salt and pepper, to taste.
5. Transfer to bowls and savor.

Nutritional Information (per serving)

Calories: 450
Fat: 15g
Protein: 15g
Carbohydrates: 65g
Fiber: 14g
Cholesterol: 0mg

Turkey and Veggie Wrap

Servings: 2
Cooking Time: 10 minutes
Prep Time: 15 minutes
Total Time: 25 minutes

Ingredients

1/2 lb ground turkey
1 tablespoon olive oil
1 bell pepper, thinly sliced
1 zucchini, julienned
1/2 cup cherry tomatoes, halved
1 teaspoon cumin
1/2 teaspoon paprika
Salt and pepper to taste
2 whole wheat wraps
1/4 cup hummus

Instructions

1. Heat the olive oil in a skillet over medium heat.
2. Add the ground turkey and use a spatula to split it up as it cooks until browned.
3. Include the bell pepper, cherry tomatoes, zucchini, paprika, cumin, and salt and pepper. Simmer for five more minutes.
4. Use a pan or microwave to reheat the whole wheat wraps.
5. Evenly distribute hummus onto every wrap.
6. Divide the vegetable and turkey mixture among the wraps.
7. Tightly roll the wraps after folding the sides.
8. Cut in half and present.

Nutritional Information (per serving)

Calories: 420
Fat: 18g
Protein: 25g
Carbohydrates: 40g
Fiber: 8g

Cholesterol: 50mg

Vegetable Stir-Fry

Servings: 4
Cooking Time: 15 minutes
Prep Time: 20 minutes
Total Time: 35 minutes

Ingredients

2 cups broccoli florets
1 bell pepper, thinly sliced
1 carrot, julienned
1 cup snap peas, trimmed
1 cup mushrooms, sliced
2 tablespoons soy sauce
1 tablespoon sesame oil
1 tablespoon ginger, minced
2 cloves garlic, minced
1 tablespoon vegetable oil
2 cups cooked brown rice

Instructions

1. Heat the vegetable oil in a wok or big pan over medium-high heat.
2. Include the snap peas, mushrooms, bell pepper, carrot, and broccoli. Cook for five to seven minutes, or until the veggies are crisp-tender.
3. Combine the sesame oil, ginger, garlic, and soy sauce in a small bowl.
4. Drizzle the veggies with the sauce, stirring to ensure uniform coating.
5. Cook for a further two to three minutes.
6. Top cooked brown rice with the stir-fried veggies.

Nutritional Information (per serving)

Calories: 280
Fat: 8g
Protein: 6g
Carbohydrates: 45g
Fiber: 6g
Cholesterol: 0mg

Salmon and Asparagus

Servings: 2
Cooking Time: 20 minutes
Prep Time: 10 minutes
Total Time: 30 minutes

Ingredients

2 salmon filets
1 bunch asparagus, trimmed
1 lemon, sliced
2 tablespoons olive oil
1 teaspoon garlic powder
Salt and pepper to taste

Instructions

1. Set the oven's temperature to 400°F, or 200°C.
2. Place the salmon filets on a baking tray lined with parchment paper.
3. Place the fish surrounded by clipped asparagus.
4. Give the asparagus and fish a drizzle of olive oil.
5. Use salt, pepper, and garlic powder to season the fish. Top with slices of lemon.
6. Bake for 15 to 18 minutes, or until a fork can easily pierce the salmon.
7. Garnish the asparagus and salmon with a squeeze of lemon juice.

Nutritional Information (per serving)

Calories: 350
Fat: 22g
Protein: 30g
Carbohydrates: 10g
Fiber: 4g
Cholesterol: 80mg

Caprese Salad

Servings: 4
Cooking Time: 10 minutes
Prep Time: 10 minutes
Total Time: 20 minutes

Ingredients

4 large tomatoes, sliced
1 ball fresh mozzarella, sliced
1 bunch fresh basil leaves
3 tablespoons balsamic glaze
2 tablespoons extra-virgin olive oil
Salt and pepper to taste

Instructions

1. On a serving dish, arrange tomato and mozzarella slices in succession.
2. Place a few fresh basil leaves in between the mozzarella and tomato slices.
3. Drizzle the salad with extra-virgin olive oil and balsamic glaze.
4. Season with salt and pepper, to taste.
5. Serve right now as a cool side dish.

Nutritional Information (per serving)

Calories: 180
Fat: 14g
Protein: 8g
Carbohydrates: 8g
Fiber: 2g
Cholesterol: 25mg

Shrimp and Broccoli Stir-Fry

Servings: 3
Cooking Time: 15 minutes
Prep Time: 10 minutes
Total Time: 25 minutes

Ingredients

1 lb shrimp, peeled and deveined
3 cups broccoli florets
1 red bell pepper, thinly sliced
2 tablespoons soy sauce
1 tablespoon hoisin sauce
1 tablespoon sesame oil
1 tablespoon vegetable oil
1 tablespoon ginger, minced
2 cloves garlic, minced
2 green onions, sliced
Sesame seeds for garnish

Instructions

1. Heat the vegetable oil in a wok or big pan over medium-high heat.
2. Stir-fry the shrimp for two to three minutes, or until they are opaque and pink. Take out of the wok and put aside.
3. Add the broccoli, red bell pepper, ginger, and garlic to the same wok. Vegetables should be stir-fried for 5 to 7 minutes to make them crisp-tender.
4. Combine the sesame oil, hoisin sauce, and soy sauce in a small bowl.
5. Return the cooked shrimp to the pan and cover the contents with the sauce.
6. Stir-fry for two to three more minutes, or until everything is well coated.
7. Add sesame seeds and sliced green onions as garnish.
8. Present with noodles or rice.

Nutritional Information (per serving)

Calories: 280g
Fat: 12g
Protein: 25g

Carbohydrates: 16g
Fiber: 4g
Cholesterol: 180mg

Mediterranean Chickpea Salad

Servings: 4
Cooking Time: 10 minutes
Prep Time: 15 minutes
Total Time: 25 minutes

Ingredients

2 cans (15 oz each) chickpeas, drained and rinsed
1 cucumber, diced
1 cup cherry tomatoes, halved
1/2 red onion, finely chopped
1/2 cup Kalamata olives, sliced
1/2 cup crumbled feta cheese
3 tablespoons extra-virgin olive oil
2 tablespoons red wine vinegar
1 teaspoon dried oregano
Salt and pepper to taste

Instructions

1. Combine the chickpeas, cucumber, red onion, cherry tomatoes, olives, and feta cheese in a big bowl.
2. Combine the olive oil, red wine vinegar, dried oregano, salt, and pepper in a small bowl.
3. Drizzle the chickpea mixture with the dressing and gently toss to coat.
4. Before serving, let the salad marinade for a few minutes.
5. Serve as a cool salad or a side dish, adjusting the flavor as necessary.

Nutritional Information (per serving)

Calories: 380
Fat: 20g
Protein: 15g
Carbohydrates: 40g
Fiber: 12g
Cholesterol: 15mg

Veggie Wrap with Hummus

Servings: 2
Cooking Time: 10 minutes
Prep Time: 15 minutes
Total Time: 25 minutes

Ingredients

2 whole wheat wraps
1 cup hummus
1 bell pepper, thinly sliced
1 cucumber, julienned
1 carrot, grated
1/2 cup cherry tomatoes, halved
1/4 cup red onion, thinly sliced
2 cups mixed salad greens

Instructions

Place a thick layer of hummus on top of every whole wheat wrap.
2. Evenly top the wraps with bell pepper, mixed salad greens, cucumber, carrot, cherry tomatoes, and red onion.
3. Tightly roll the wraps, tucking in the edges as you roll.
4. Before serving, cut in half diagonally.

Nutritional Information (per serving)

Calories: 320
Fat: 14g
Protein: 10g
Carbohydrates: 45g
Fiber: 10g
Cholesterol: 0mg

Tuna Salad Lettuce Wraps

Servings: 4
Cooking Time: 10 minutes
Prep Time: 15 minutes
Total Time: 25 minutes

Ingredients

2 cans (5 oz each) tuna, drained
- 1/4 cup mayonnaise
2 tablespoons Greek yogurt
1 celery stalk, finely diced
1/4 cup red onion, finely chopped
1 tablespoon Dijon mustard
Salt and pepper to taste
8 large lettuce leaves

Instructions

1. Put the tuna, Greek yogurt, mayonnaise, celery, red onion, Dijon mustard, salt, and pepper in a bowl.
2. Thoroughly combine the ingredients by mixing them.
3. Evenly distribute the tuna salad across big lettuce leaves using a spoon.
4. Encircle the tuna salad in the lettuce, tying it off with toothpicks if necessary.
5. Serve right away as a filling and light lunch or snack.

Nutritional Information (per serving)

Calories: 180
Fat: 10g
Protein: 20g
Carbohydrates: 4g
Fiber: 1g
Cholesterol: 25mg

Sweet Potato and Black Bean Bowl

Servings: 2
Cooking Time: 25 minutes
Prep Time: 15 minutes
Total Time: 40 minutes

Ingredients

2 medium sweet potatoes, peeled and diced
One can (15 oz) of rinsed and drained black beans
1 cup corn kernels
1 avocado, sliced
1/4 cup cilantro, chopped
2 tablespoons lime juice
1 tablespoon olive oil
1 teaspoon ground cumin
Salt and pepper to taste

Instructions

1. Set the oven's temperature to 400°F, or 200°C.
2. Combine olive oil, cumin, salt, and pepper with chopped sweet potatoes.
3. Bake sweet potatoes for 20 to 25 minutes on a baking sheet, or until they are soft and beginning to crisp up.
4. Combine corn, black beans, avocado, cilantro, and lime juice in a bowl.
5. Gently toss in the cooked sweet potatoes after adding them to the mixture.
6. Make any necessary seasoning adjustments and serve as a filling bowl.

Nutritional Information (per serving)

Calories: 380
Fat: 15g
Protein: 10g
Carbohydrates: 55g
Fiber: 14g
Cholesterol: 0mg

Chicken Caesar Salad

Servings: 4
Cooking Time: 15 minutes
Prep Time: 15 minutes
Total Time: 30 minutes

Ingredients

2 boneless, skinless chicken breasts
1 head romaine lettuce, chopped
1 cup cherry tomatoes, halved
1/2 cup croutons
1/2 cup grated Parmesan cheese
1/4 cup Caesar dressing
1 tablespoon olive oil
Salt and pepper to taste

Instructions

1. Sprinkle salt and pepper on the chicken breasts.
2. In a pan over medium-high heat, warm the olive oil.
3. Cook chicken until cooked through, 6 to 8 minutes each side.
4. Give the chicken five minutes to rest before slicing.
5. Put the chopped romaine lettuce, cherry tomatoes, croutons, and Parmesan cheese in a big bowl.
6. Place chicken slices on top.
7. Cover the salad with a drizzle of Caesar dressing and gently toss to coat.
8. For a traditional and filling Caesar salad, serve right away.

Nutritional Information (per serving)

Calories: 350
Fat: 18g
Protein: 30g
Carbohydrates: 20g
Fiber: 4g
Cholesterol: 80mg

Quinoa Stuffed Peppers

Servings: 4
Cooking Time: 40 minutes
Prep Time: 20 minutes
Total Time: 1 hour

Ingredients

Four big bell peppers, seeded and halved
1 cup quinoa, rinsed
2 cups vegetable broth
One can (15 oz) of rinsed and drained black beans
1 cup corn kernels
1 cup cherry tomatoes, diced
1/2 cup red onion, finely chopped
1 teaspoon cumin
1 teaspoon chili powder
Salt and pepper to taste
1 cup shredded cheddar cheese (optional)
Fresh cilantro for garnish

Instructions

Set the oven's temperature to 375°F, or 190°C.
2. Put the quinoa and vegetable broth in a saucepan. After bringing to a boil, lower the heat, cover, and simmer the quinoa for 15 minutes, or until it is tender.
3. Combine cooked quinoa, black beans, corn, red onion, cherry tomatoes, cumin, chili powder, salt, and pepper in a big bowl.
4. Put the halves of the bell pepper in a baking tray.
The quinoa mixture should be spooned into each pepper half.
6. You may top with shredded cheddar cheese, if you'd like.
7. Bake the peppers for 25 to 30 minutes, or until they are soft.
8. Before serving, garnish with fresh cilantro.

Nutritional Information (per serving)

Calories: 380
Fat: 10g
Protein: 15g

Carbohydrates: 60g
Fiber: 10g
Cholesterol: 20mg

Lentil Soup

Servings: 6
Cooking Time: 45 minutes
Prep Time: 15 minutes
Total Time: 1 hour

Ingredients

One cup of washed and dried green or brown lentils
1 onion, finely chopped
2 carrots, diced
2 celery stalks, diced
3 cloves garlic, minced
1 can (14 oz) diced tomatoes
6 cups vegetable broth
1 teaspoon ground cumin
1 teaspoon smoked paprika
1/2 teaspoon dried thyme
Salt and pepper to taste
2 cups spinach or kale, chopped
Lemon wedges for serving

Instructions

1. In a big saucepan, cook the celery, carrots, and onions over medium heat until they are tender.
2. Cook the minced garlic for one to two more minutes.
3. Add the diced tomatoes, cumin, smoky paprika, thyme, vegetable broth, lentils, and salt and pepper.
4. After bringing the soup to a boil, lower the heat, and simmer it until the lentils are soft, around 30 to 35 minutes.
5. Cook for a further five minutes after adding the chopped kale or spinach.
6. Taste and adjust seasoning.
7. Garnish with freshly squeezed lemon juice and serve hot.

Nutritional Information (per serving)

Calories: 220
Fat: 1g
Protein: 14g

Carbohydrates: 40g
Fiber: 12g
Cholesterol: 0mg

Turkey and Quinoa Meatballs

Servings: 4
Cooking Time: 25 minutes
Prep Time: 20 minutes
Total Time: 45 minutes

Ingredients

1 lb ground turkey
1 cup cooked quinoa
1/2 cup breadcrumbs
1/4 cup grated Parmesan cheese
1 egg
2 cloves garlic, minced
1 teaspoon dried oregano
1/2 teaspoon onion powder
Salt and pepper to taste
2 cups marinara sauce
Fresh parsley for garnish

Instructions

1. Set the oven's temperature to 400°F, or 200°C.
2. Combine the cooked quinoa, ground turkey, breadcrumbs, Parmesan cheese, egg, garlic, oregano, onion powder, salt, and pepper in a big bowl.
3. Form into meatballs by mixing well.
4. Transfer meatballs to a parchment paper-lined baking sheet.
5. Bake until cooked through, 20 to 25 minutes.
6. Heat the marinara sauce in a skillet over medium heat.
7. Simmer the cooked meatballs in the sauce for five minutes.
8. Before serving, garnish with fresh parsley.

Nutritional Information (per serving)

Calories: 320
Fat: 15g
Protein: 25g
Carbohydrates: 20g

Fiber: 3g
Cholesterol: 110mg

Veggie Wrap with Avocado

Servings: 2
Cooking Time: 10 minutes
Prep Time: 15 minutes
Total Time: 25 minutes

Ingredients

2 whole wheat wraps
1 ripe avocado, mashed
1 cup hummus
1 bell pepper, thinly sliced
1 cucumber, julienned
1 carrot, grated
1/4 cup red onion, thinly sliced
2 cups mixed salad greens

Instructions

1. Toast each whole wheat wrapper and top with a layer of mashed avocado.
2. Evenly top the wraps with hummus, mixed salad leaves, bell pepper, cucumber, carrot, and red onion.
3. Tightly roll the wraps, tucking in the edges as you roll.
4. Before serving, cut in half diagonally.

Nutritional Information (per serving)

Calories: 340
Fat: 15g
Protein: 10g
Carbohydrates: 45g
Fiber: 10g
Cholesterol: 0mg

Pesto Zoodles with Cherry Tomatoes

Servings: 2
Cooking Time: 15 minutes
Prep Time: 10 minutes
Total Time: 25 minutes

Ingredients

4 medium zucchinis, spiralized into zoodles
1 cup cherry tomatoes, halved
1/4 cup pine nuts, toasted
1/2 cup fresh basil leaves
2 cloves garlic
1/3 cup grated Parmesan cheese
1/3 cup extra-virgin olive oil
Salt and pepper to taste

Instructions

1. Put the pine nuts, Parmesan cheese, fresh basil, and garlic in a food processor or blender.
2. Pulse until chopped finely.
3. Add olive oil to the pesto gradually while the blender is running, until it is smooth.
4. Sauté the zoodles in a large pan over medium heat for 3–4 minutes, or until they are just soft.
5. Cook for a further two minutes after adding the cherry tomatoes.
6. Add the prepared pesto and toss to evenly cover the tomatoes and zoodles.
7. To taste, add salt and pepper for seasoning.
8. Present right away, topped with more pine nuts and Parmesan, if preferred.

Nutritional Information (per serving)

Calories: 350
Fat: 30g
Protein: 10g
Carbohydrates: 15g
Fiber: 5g
Cholesterol: 10mg

Chickpea and Spinach Salad

Servings: 4
Cooking Time: 10 minutes
Prep Time: 15 minutes
Total Time: 25 minutes

Ingredients

2 cans (15 oz each) chickpeas, drained and rinsed
4 cups fresh spinach leaves
1 cup cherry tomatoes, halved
1/2 cucumber, diced
1/4 cup red onion, finely chopped
1/3 cup feta cheese, crumbled
2 tablespoons extra-virgin olive oil
2 tablespoons balsamic vinegar
1 teaspoon Dijon mustard
Salt and pepper to taste

Instructions

1. Put the chickpeas, feta cheese, cherry tomatoes, cucumber, red onion, and fresh spinach in a big bowl.
2. Combine the olive oil, balsamic vinegar, Dijon mustard, salt, and pepper in a small bowl.
3. Pour the salad with the dressing and gently toss to coat.
4. Give the salad a few minutes to settle so the flavors can combine.
5. Serve as a colorful and nourishing salad, adjusting the flavor as required.

Nutritional Information (per serving)

Calories: 320
Fat: 15g
Protein: 12g
Carbohydrates: 40g
Fiber: 10g
Cholesterol: 10mg

Cauliflower Fried Rice

Servings: 4
Cooking Time: 20 minutes
Prep Time: 15 minutes
Total Time: 35 minutes

Ingredients

1 medium cauliflower, riced
2 tablespoons vegetable oil
1 cup frozen peas and carrots, thawed
2 green onions, sliced
3 cloves garlic, minced
2 eggs, beaten
3 tablespoons soy sauce
1 teaspoon sesame oil
1/2 teaspoon ginger, grated
Sesame seeds and chopped cilantro for garnish

Instructions

1. Pulse the cauliflower in a food processor until the chunks resemble rice.
2. Heat vegetable oil in a big pan over medium heat.
3. Include the garlic, green onions, carrots, and peas. Cook the veggies for 3–4 minutes, or until they become soft.
4. Transfer veggies to one side of the pan and transfer the beaten eggs to the other.
5. After the eggs are fully cooked, scramble them and combine them with the veggies.
6. Add the riced cauliflower to the pan and mix everything together.
7. Combine the grated ginger, sesame oil, and soy sauce in a small bowl.
8. Drizzle the cauliflower mixture with the sauce, then toss to ensure uniform coating.
9. Cook until the cauliflower is soft, about 5 to 7 more minutes.
10. Before serving, garnish with chopped cilantro and sesame seeds.

Nutritional Information (per serving)

Calories: 180
Fat: 10g
Protein: 8g
Carbohydrates: 15g

Fiber: 5g
Cholesterol: 95mg

Egg Salad Lettuce Wraps

Servings: 4
Cooking Time: 10 minutes
Prep Time: 10 minutes
Total Time: 20 minutes

Ingredients

6 hard-boiled eggs, chopped
1/4 cup mayonnaise
1 tablespoon Dijon mustard
2 green onions, finely sliced
1 celery stalk, finely diced
Salt and pepper to taste
8 large lettuce leaves

Instructions

1. Combine chopped hard-boiled eggs, green onions, celery, mayonnaise, Dijon mustard, and salt and pepper in a bowl.
2. Continue stirring until all of the ingredients are combined.
3. Transfer the egg salad over broad leaf lettuce.
4. Encircle the egg salad in the lettuce, tying it off with toothpicks if necessary.
5. Serve right away as a filling and light lunch or snack.

Nutritional Information (per serving)

Calories: 220
Fat: 18g
Protein: 10g
Carbohydrates: 2g
Fiber: 1g
Cholesterol: 280mg

Blackened Chicken Salad

Servings: 4
Cooking Time: 20 minutes
Prep Time: 15 minutes
Total Time: 35 minutes

Ingredients

4 boneless, skinless chicken breasts
2 tablespoons blackened seasoning
2 tablespoons olive oil
8 cups mixed salad greens
1 cup cherry tomatoes, halved
1 cucumber, sliced
1/2 red onion, thinly sliced
1/4 cup crumbled blue cheese
1/4 cup balsamic vinaigrette dressing

Instructions

1. Evenly coat each chicken breast with the blackened seasoning.
2. In a pan over medium-high heat, warm the olive oil.
3. Cook chicken until cooked through, 6 to 8 minutes each side.
4. Give the chicken five minutes to rest before slicing.
5. Combine salad greens, cucumber, red onion, cherry tomatoes, and crumbled blue cheese in a big bowl.
6. Place sliced charred chicken on top of the salad.
7. Cover the salad with a balsamic vinaigrette dressing.
8. Gently toss to mix and proceed to serve.

Nutritional Information (per serving)

Calories: 320
Fat: 15g
Protein: 30g
Carbohydrates: 15g
Fiber: 4g
Cholesterol: 80mg

Chapter 5: Dinner Delights

Baked Cod with Lemon and Herbs

Servings: 4
Cooking Time: 20 minutes
Prep Time: 10 minutes
Total Time: 30 minutes

Ingredients

4 cod filets
2 tablespoons olive oil
1 lemon (sliced)
2 teaspoons fresh thyme (chopped)
2 teaspoons fresh rosemary (chopped)
Salt and pepper to taste

Instructions

1. Set the oven's temperature to 400°F, or 200°C.
2. Put the filets of fish onto a roasting dish.
3. Add lemon slices, drizzle with olive oil, and season with salt, pepper, thyme, and rosemary.
4. Bake the fish for 20 minutes, or until it is well done.

Nutritional Information

Calories: 250
Fat: 10g
Protein: 30g
Carbohydrates: 3g
Cholesterol: 70mg

Vegetarian Chili

Servings: 6
Cooking Time: 40 minutes
Prep Time: 15 minutes
Total Time: 55 minutes

Ingredients

2 cans (15 oz each) black beans (drained and rinsed)
1 can (15 oz) kidney beans (drained and rinsed)
1 can (15 oz) diced tomatoes
1 cup corn kernels (frozen or fresh)
1 onion (diced)
2 bell peppers (diced)
3 cloves garlic (minced)
2 tablespoons chili powder
1 tablespoon cumin
Salt and pepper to taste

Instructions

1. Saute the garlic, bell peppers, and onions in a big saucepan until they become tender.
2. Include the tomatoes, beans, corn, cumin, chili powder, salt, and pepper.
3. Simmer for half an hour.

Nutritional Information

Calories: 300
Fat: 1g
Protein: 15g
Carbohydrates: 60g
Cholesterol: 0mg

Teriyaki Tofu Stir-Fry

Servings: 4
Cooking Time: 15 minutes
Prep Time: 10 minutes
Total Time: 25 minutes

Ingredients

1 block firm tofu (cubed)
2 cups broccoli florets
1 bell pepper (sliced)
1 carrot (julienned)
1/4 cup teriyaki sauce
2 tablespoons soy sauce
1 tablespoon sesame oil
1 tablespoon ginger (minced)
2 cloves garlic (minced)

Instructions

1. After pressing the tofu to get rid of extra water, stir-fry it till golden brown.
2. Continue stir-frying after adding the broccoli, bell pepper, and carrot.
3. Combine the sesame oil, ginger, garlic, soy sauce, and teriyaki sauce in a bowl.
4. Drizzle the tofu and veggies with the sauce, stirring to coat.

Nutritional Information

Calories: 280
Fat: 15g
Protein: 20g
Carbohydrates: 25g
Cholesterol: 0mg

Pesto Chicken and Veggie Skewers

Servings: 4
Cooking Time: 20 minutes
Prep Time: 15 minutes
Total Time: 35 minutes

Ingredients

1 lb chicken breast (cut into chunks)
1 zucchini (sliced)
1 bell pepper (sliced)
1/2 cup cherry tomatoes
1/4 cup pesto sauce
Salt and pepper to taste

Instructions

1. Thread tomatoes, bell pepper, zucchini, and chicken onto skewers.
2. Add salt and pepper for seasoning, then drizzle with pesto.
3. Cook the chicken thoroughly on the grill or in the oven.

Nutritional Information

Calories: 320
Fat: 12g
Protein: 30g
Carbohydrates: 15g
Cholesterol: 80mg

Spaghetti Squash with Marinara

Servings: 2
Cooking Time: 45 minutes
Prep Time: 10 minutes
Total Time: 55 minutes

Ingredients

1 medium-sized spaghetti squash
2 cups marinara sauce
1 tablespoon olive oil
2 cloves garlic (minced)
1 teaspoon dried oregano
Salt and pepper to taste

Instructions

1. Halve the spaghetti squash, scrape out the seeds, and bake until soft.
2. Add oregano, marinara sauce, salt, and pepper to a skillet with sautéed garlic in olive oil.
3. Scrape the cooked squash into "spaghetti" strands with a fork.
4. Drizzle spaghetti squash strands with marinara sauce.

Nutritional Information

Calories: 180
Fat: 5g
Protein: 3g
Carbohydrates: 30g
Cholesterol: 0mg

Salmon and Quinoa Salad

Servings: 3
Cooking Time: 20 minutes
Prep Time: 15 minutes
Total Time: 35 minutes

Ingredients

1 cup quinoa (cooked)
1 lb salmon filets (grilled and flaked)
1 cup cherry tomatoes (halved)
1 cucumber (diced)
1/4 cup red onion (finely chopped)
2 tablespoons olive oil
1 tablespoon balsamic vinegar
Salt and pepper to taste

Instructions

1. Combine the quinoa, cucumber, red onion, cherry tomatoes, and grilled salmon in a bowl.
2. Add a balsamic vinegar and olive oil drizzle, then season with salt and pepper.
3. Gently toss to mix.

Nutritional Information

Calories: 350
Fat: 18g
Protein: 25g
Carbohydrates: 25g
Cholesterol: 60mg

Stuffed Bell Peppers with Turkey

Servings: 5
Cooking Time: 40 minutes
Prep Time: 20 minutes
Total Time: 1 hour

Ingredients

5 bell peppers (halved and seeds removed)
1 lb ground turkey
1 cup cooked brown rice
1 can (15 oz) black beans (drained and rinsed)
1 cup corn kernels (frozen or fresh)
1 cup tomato sauce
1 teaspoon cumin
1 teaspoon chili powder
Salt and pepper to taste

Instructions

1. Set oven temperature to 190°C/375°F.
2. Cook the ground turkey in a pan until browned.
3. Combine the turkey with the cooked rice, tomato sauce, black beans, corn, chili powder, cumin, and salt and pepper.
4. Stuff the mixture into each side of a bell pepper.
5. Bake for an hour and a half.

Nutritional Information

Calories: 320
Fat: 10g
Protein: 20g
Carbohydrates: 40g
Cholesterol: 50mg

Lemon Garlic Shrimp Pasta

Servings: 4
Cooking Time: 15 minutes
Prep Time: 10 minutes
Total Time: 25 minutes

Ingredients

8 oz linguine or your preferred pasta
1 lb large shrimp (peeled and deveined)
3 tablespoons olive oil
4 cloves garlic (minced)
Zest of 1 lemon
Juice of 1 lemon
1/4 cup fresh parsley (chopped)
Salt and pepper to taste

Instructions

1. Prepare pasta as directed on the box.
2. Sauté shrimp in olive oil in a skillet until they become pink.
3. Include the lemon juice, garlic, and zest. Simmer for a further two to three minutes.
4. Combine the shrimp mixture with the cooked pasta.
5. Sprinkle some fresh parsley on top and add some salt and pepper to taste.

Nutritional Information

Calories: 400
Fat: 12g
Protein: 25g
Carbohydrates: 50g
Cholesterol: 150mg

Eggplant Parmesan

Servings: 6
Cooking Time: 45 minutes
Prep Time: 20 minutes
Total Time: 1 hour and 5 minutes

Ingredients

2 medium-sized eggplants (sliced)
2 cups marinara sauce
2 cups mozzarella cheese (shredded)
1 cup Parmesan cheese (grated)
1 cup breadcrumbs
2 eggs (beaten)
1/4 cup fresh basil (chopped)
Salt and pepper to taste

Instructions

1. Set oven temperature to 190°C/375°F.
2. Coat bread crumbs on eggplant slices after dipping them in beaten eggs.
3. Bake slices of eggplant until they get golden brown.
4. Arrange the eggplant, mozzarella, Parmesan, and marinara sauce in a baking dish.
5. Continue layering, and then top with cheese.
6. Bake until bubbling and golden, 25 to 30 minutes.

Nutritional Information

Calories: 320
Fat: 15g
Protein: 20g
Carbohydrates: 25g
Cholesterol: 70mg

Cauliflower Pizza Crust

Servings: 2 (1 pizza)
Cooking Time: 25 minutes
Prep Time: 15 minutes
Total Time: 40 minutes

Ingredients

1 small cauliflower head (riced)
1 cup mozzarella cheese (shredded)
1 egg
1 teaspoon dried oregano
1 teaspoon garlic powder
Salt and pepper to taste

Instructions

1. Set oven temperature to 200°C/400°F.
2. After 5 minutes of microwave cooking, let the riced cauliflower cool and then wring out any extra liquid.
3. Combine the cauliflower, egg, garlic powder, oregano, salt, and pepper with the mozzarella.
4. Using a baking sheet, spread the ingredients to create a pizza crust.
5. Bake until golden, about 20 minutes.
6. Top pizza with preferred ingredients and bake until cheese is melted.

Nutritional Information

Calories: 180
Fat: 10g
Protein: 15g
Carbohydrates: 15g
Cholesterol: 80mg

Turkey and Sweet Potato Skillet

Servings: 4
Cooking Time: 30 minutes
Prep Time: 15 minutes
Total Time: 45 minutes

Ingredients

1 lb ground turkey
2 sweet potatoes (peeled and diced)
1 onion (diced)
1 bell pepper (diced)
2 cloves garlic (minced)
1 teaspoon cumin
1 teaspoon smoked paprika
Salt and pepper to taste
2 tablespoons olive oil

Instruction

1. Heat the olive oil in a big pan and sauté the garlic and onions.
2. Add the turkey meat and heat it until browned.
3. Include the smoked paprika, bell pepper, cumin, sweet potatoes, salt, and pepper.
4. Cook the sweet potatoes covered until they are soft.

Nutritional Information

Calories: 350
Fat: 15g
Protein: 25g
Carbohydrates: 30g
Cholesterol: 60mg

Sesame Ginger Salmon

Servings: 2
Cooking Time: 15 minutes
Prep Time: 10 minutes
Total Time: 25 minutes

Ingredients

2 salmon filets
2 tablespoons soy sauce
1 tablespoon sesame oil
1 tablespoon rice vinegar
1 tablespoon honey
1 teaspoon fresh ginger (grated)
1 teaspoon sesame seeds

Instructions

1. Set the oven's temperature to 400°F, or 200°C.
2. Combine soy sauce, rice vinegar, honey, sesame oil, and grated ginger in a bowl.
3. Lay out the salmon filets and drizzle with the sauce on a baking pan.
4. Bake the salmon for 12 to 15 minutes, or until it is done.
5. Before serving, top with sesame seeds.

Nutritional Information

Calories: 300
Fat: 15g
Protein: 25g
Carbohydrates: 15g
Cholesterol: 60mg

Chickpea and Spinach Curry

Servings: 4
Cooking Time: 25 minutes
Prep Time: 10 minutes
Total Time: 35 minutes

Ingredients

Two cans (15 oz each) of rinsed and drained chickpeas
1 onion (finely chopped)
2 tomatoes (diced)
3 cups fresh spinach leaves
2 tablespoons curry powder
1 teaspoon cumin
1 teaspoon coriander
1 teaspoon turmeric
1/2 cup coconut milk
Salt and pepper to taste

Instructions

1. Saute onions in a pan until they get yellow.
2. Add the curry powder, cumin, coriander, turmeric, tomatoes, chickpeas, salt, and pepper.
3. After adding the coconut milk, simmer for fifteen minutes.
4. Cook the fresh spinach until it wilts.

Nutritional Information

Calories: 300
Fat: 8g
Protein: 15g
Carbohydrates: 45g
Cholesterol: 0mg

Mushroom and Spinach Stuffed Chicken

Servings: 2
Cooking Time: 30 minutes
Prep Time: 15 minutes
Total Time: 45 minutes

Ingredients

2 boneless, skinless chicken breasts
1 cup mushrooms (sliced)
1 cup fresh spinach
1/2 cup feta cheese (crumbled)
2 cloves garlic (minced)
2 tablespoons olive oil
Salt and pepper to taste

Instructions

1. Set oven temperature to 190°C/375°F.
2. Use salt and pepper to season chicken breasts and butterfly them.
3. Sauté garlic and mushrooms in olive oil in a skillet until they are soft.
4. Stir in feta after adding fresh spinach and mixing until it wilts.
5. Stuff the combination of mushrooms and spinach into each chicken breast.
6. Bake the chicken for 25 to 30 minutes, or until it is well done.

Nutritional Information

Calories: 400
Fat: 20g
Protein: 40g
Carbohydrates: 10g
Cholesterol: 120mg

Quinoa and Vegetable Stir-Fry

Servings: 4
Cooking Time: 20 minutes
Prep Time: 15 minutes
Total Time: 35 minutes

Ingredients

1 cup quinoa (uncooked)
2 cups broccoli florets
1 bell pepper (sliced)
1 carrot (julienned)
1 cup snap peas
3 tablespoons soy sauce
1 tablespoon sesame oil
1 tablespoon rice vinegar
1 teaspoon ginger (minced)
2 cloves garlic (minced)

Instructions

1. Prepare the quinoa per the directions on the box.
2. Stir-fry the broccoli, bell pepper, carrot, and snap peas in a wok or big pan.
3. Combine the rice vinegar, ginger, garlic, sesame oil, and soy sauce in a small bowl.
4. Stir-fry the veggies with the cooked quinoa and sauce until well mixed.

Nutritional Information

Calories: 350
Fat: 10g
Protein: 15g
Carbohydrates: 50g
Cholesterol: 0mg

Sweet Potato and Black Bean Enchiladas

Servings: 6
Cooking Time: 40 minutes
Prep Time: 20 minutes
Total Time: 1 hour

Ingredients

2 large sweet potatoes (peeled and diced)
1 can (15 oz) black beans (drained and rinsed)
1 cup corn kernels (frozen or fresh)
1 onion (diced)
1 teaspoon cumin
1 teaspoon chili powder
1/2 teaspoon paprika
12 small corn tortillas
2 cups enchilada sauce
1 cup shredded cheddar cheese

Instructions

1. Set oven temperature to 190°C/375°F.
2. After sweet potatoes are soft, boil them and mash them.
3. Add black beans, corn, cumin, chili powder, and paprika to a skillet with sautéed onions.
4. Stuff each tortilla with the bean mixture and mashed sweet potatoes, wrap it up, and put it in a baking tray.
5. Drizzle the tortillas with enchilada sauce and top with cheese.
6. Bake the cheese for 25 to 30 minutes, or until it melts and bubbles.

Nutritional Information

Calories: 400
Fat: 15g
Protein: 15g
Carbohydrates: 55g
Cholesterol: 30mg

Lemon Herb Grilled Shrimp

Servings: 4
Cooking Time: 10 minutes
Prep Time: 15 minutes
Total Time: 25 minutes

Ingredients

1 lb large shrimp (peeled and deveined)
2 tablespoons olive oil
Zest and juice of 2 lemons
2 tablespoons fresh parsley (chopped)
1 teaspoon dried oregano
1 teaspoon garlic powder
Salt and pepper to taste

Instructions

1. Combine olive oil, lemon juice, zest, parsley, oregano, garlic powder, salt, and pepper in a bowl.
2. After tossing the shrimp, cover and allow marinate for ten minutes.
3. After skewering the shrimp, grill them for two to three minutes on each side, or until done.

Nutritional Information

Calories: 180
Fat: 10g
Protein: 20g
Carbohydrates: 2g
Cholesterol: 180mg

Turkey and Veggie Skillet

Servings: 4
Cooking Time: 25 minutes
Prep Time: 15 minutes
Total Time: 40 minutes

Ingredients

1 lb ground turkey
1 zucchini (sliced)
1 bell pepper (sliced)
1 cup cherry tomatoes (halved)
1 onion (diced)
2 cloves garlic (minced)
1 teaspoon Italian seasoning
Salt and pepper to taste
2 tablespoons olive oil

Instructions

1. Cook the ground turkey in a pan until browned.
2. Add the garlic, onions, and olive oil; sauté until the garlic is tender.
3. Include the zucchini, cherry tomatoes, bell pepper, Italian seasoning, salt, and pepper.
4. Simmer the veggies for tenderness.

Nutritional Information

Calories: 320
Fat: 15g
Protein: 25g
Carbohydrates: 20g
Cholesterol: 80mg

Zucchini Noodles with Pesto

Servings: 2
Cooking Time: 15 minutes
Prep Time: 10 minutes
Total Time: 25 minutes

Ingredients

2 large zucchinis (spiralized into noodles)
1/2 cup cherry tomatoes (halved)
1/4 cup pine nuts (toasted)
1/2 cup fresh basil leaves
1/4 cup Parmesan cheese (grated)
2 cloves garlic (minced)
1/3 cup extra virgin olive oil
Salt and pepper to taste

Instructions

1. Put the garlic, basil, pine nuts, Parmesan, salt, and pepper in a food processor or blender.
2. Gradually add olive oil while mixing to create a creamy pesto sauce.
3. Sauté zucchini noodles in a skillet until they are slightly soft.
4. Combine the noodles with the ready-made pesto sauce and cherry tomatoes.

Nutritional Information

Calories: 300
Fat: 25g
Protein: 8g
Carbohydrates: 15g
Cholesterol: 5mg

Baked Chicken with Rosemary and Lemon

Servings: 4
Cooking Time: 40 minutes
Prep Time: 15 minutes
Total Time: 55 minutes

Ingredients

4 boneless, skinless chicken breasts
2 tablespoons olive oil
Zest and juice of 1 lemon
2 tablespoons fresh rosemary (chopped)
3 cloves garlic (minced)
Salt and pepper to taste

Instructions

1. Set oven temperature to 190°C/375°F.
2. Season chicken breasts with salt, pepper, rosemary, garlic, lemon zest, and lemon juice using olive oil.
3. Put the chicken in the oven for 35 to 40 minutes, or until it is cooked through.

Nutritional Information

Calories: 280
Fat: 12g
Protein: 30g
Carbohydrates: 3g
Cholesterol: 80mg

Vegetable and Quinoa Stuffed Portobello Mushrooms

Servings: 3
Cooking Time: 30 minutes
Prep Time: 20 minutes
Total Time: 50 minutes

Ingredients

Three huge Portobello mushrooms (stems removed and cleaned)
1 cup quinoa (cooked)
1 zucchini (diced)
1 bell pepper (diced)
1 cup cherry tomatoes (halved)
1/2 cup feta cheese (crumbled)
2 tablespoons olive oil
1 teaspoon dried oregano
Salt and pepper to taste

Instructions

1. Set oven temperature to 190°C/375°F.
2. In a skillet, soften the bell pepper, cherry tomatoes, and zucchini by sautéing them in olive oil.
3. Combine sautéed veggies with cooked quinoa, feta, oregano, salt, and pepper.
4. Stuff the quinoa mixture into portobello mushrooms.
5. Bake until the mushrooms are soft, 20 to 25 minutes.

Nutritional Information

Calories: 300
Fat: 15g
Protein: 12g
Carbohydrates: 35g
Cholesterol: 20mg

Chapter 6: Snacks and Appetizers

Guacamole with Veggie Sticks

Servings: 4
Cooking Time: 0 minutes
Prep Time: 10 minutes
Total Time: 10 minutes

Ingredients

3 ripe avocados, mashed
1 small onion, finely diced
1 tomato, diced
1 clove garlic, minced
1 lime, juiced
Salt and pepper to taste
Assorted veggie sticks (carrots, celery, bell peppers)

Instructions

1. Combine mashed avocados, lime juice, sliced onion, tomato, and minced garlic in a bowl.
2. Add pepper and salt, and thoroughly combine.
3. Accompany guacamole with a variety of vegetable sticks.

Nutritional Information

Calories: 160 per serving
Fat: 14g
Protein: 2g
Carbohydrates: 10g
Vitamin C: 14mg
Cholesterol: 0mg

Greek Yogurt and Berry Parfait

Servings: 2
Cooking Time: 0 minutes
Prep Time: 5 minutes
Total Time: 5 minutes

Ingredients

1 cup Greek yogurt
1 cup mixed berries (strawberries, blueberries, raspberries)
2 tablespoons honey
Granola for layering

Instructions

1. Arrange Greek yogurt, granola, and mixed berries in serving glasses.
2. Pour honey on top of every layer.
3. Continue layering, and then top with a dollop of yogurt.

Nutritional Information

Calories: 250 per serving
Fat: 7g
Protein: 15g
Carbohydrates: 35g
Vitamin C: 18mg
Cholesterol: 10mg

Hummus and Veggie Platter

Servings: 6
Cooking Time: 0 minutes
Prep Time: 10 minutes
Total Time: 10 minutes

Ingredients

2 cups hummus
Assorted veggies (cucumber, cherry tomatoes, baby carrots)
Olive oil for drizzling
Paprika for garnish

Instructions

1. Spoon hummus onto a dish, centering it.
2. Cover it with a variety of vegetables.
3. Drizzle paprika on top of the hummus, drizzle with olive oil, and serve.

Nutritional Information

Calories: 180 per serving
Fat: 10g
Protein: 6g
Carbohydrates: 18g
Vitamin C: 10mg
Cholesterol: 0mg

Cottage Cheese and Pineapple Salsa

Servings: 4
Cooking Time: 0 minutes
Prep Time: 15 minutes
Total Time: 15 minutes

Ingredients

2 cups cottage cheese
1 cup fresh pineapple, diced
1/4 red onion, finely chopped
1 jalapeño, seeded and minced
2 tablespoons cilantro, chopped

Instructions

1. Combine cottage cheese, chopped red onion, jalapeño, chopped pineapple, and cilantro in a bowl.
2. Let cool for a little before serving.

Nutritional Information

Calories: 120 per serving
Fat: 3g
Protein: 14g
Carbohydrates: 12g
Vitamin C: 20mg
Cholesterol: 15mg

Baked Sweet Potato Fries

Servings: 4
Cooking Time: 25 minutes
Prep Time: 10 minutes
Total Time: 35 minutes

Ingredients

4 medium sweet potatoes, cut into fries
2 tablespoons olive oil
1 teaspoon paprika
1/2 teaspoon garlic powder
Salt and pepper to taste

Instructions

1. Set oven temperature to 425°F (220°C).
2. Combine the sweet potato fries, olive oil, salt, pepper, paprika, and garlic powder in a basin.
3. Evenly spread out on a baking sheet; bake, rotating halfway through, for 25 minutes.

Nutritional Information

Calories: 180 per serving
Fat: 7g
Protein: 2g
Carbohydrates: 30g
Vitamin A: 200% DV
Cholesterol: 0mg

Caprese Skewers

Servings: 6
Cooking Time: 0 minutes
Prep Time: 15 minutes
Total Time: 15 minutes

Ingredients

18 cherry tomatoes
18 small fresh mozzarella balls
18 fresh basil leaves
Balsamic glaze for drizzling

Instructions

1. Thread each skewer with a tomato, mozzarella ball, and basil leaf.
2. Before serving, arrange the skewers on a dish and pour balsamic glaze over them.

Nutritional Information

Calories: 120 per serving
Fat: 8g
Protein: 6g
Carbohydrates: 6g
Vitamin C: 15mg
Cholesterol: 20mg

Edamame with Sea Salt

Servings: 4
Cooking Time: 5 minutes
Prep Time: 5 minutes
Total Time: 10 minutes

Ingredients

2 cups edamame, steamed
Sea salt to taste

Instructions

1. Follow the directions on the package to steam the edamame.
2. Before serving, throw in a little sea salt.

Nutritional Information

Calories: 100 per serving
Fat: 3g
Protein: 9g
Carbohydrates: 8g
Fiber: 4g
Cholesterol: 0mg

Apple Slices with Almond Butter

Servings: 2
Cooking Time: 0 minutes
Prep Time: 5 minutes
Total Time: 5 minutes

Ingredients

2 apples, sliced
4 tablespoons almond butter

Instructions

1. Arrange slices of apple on a platter.
2. Provide almond butter on the side for dipping.

Nutritional Information

Calories: 200 per serving
Fat: 14g
Protein: 4g
Carbohydrates: 20g
Fiber: 6g
Cholesterol: 0mg

Kale Chips

Servings: 4
Cooking Time: 15 minutes
Prep Time: 10 minutes
Total Time: 25 minutes

Ingredients

One bundle of chopped and separated kale leaves
2 tablespoons olive oil
Salt and pepper to taste

Instructions

1. Set oven temperature to 175°C/350°F.
2. Combine salt, pepper, and olive oil with the kale pieces in a bowl.
3. Transfer to a baking sheet and bake until crispy, about 15 minutes.

Nutritional Information

Calories: 50 per serving
Fat: 3g
Protein: 2g
Carbohydrates: 5g
Vitamin A: 200% DV
Cholesterol: 0mg

Vegetable Spring Rolls

Servings: 8
Cooking Time: 0 minutes
Prep Time: 20 minutes
Total Time: 20 minutes

Ingredients

8 rice paper wrappers
2 cups mixed veggies (carrots, cucumber, bell peppers)
1 cup cooked vermicelli noodles
Hoisin sauce for dipping

Instructions

1. To make rice paper wrappers malleable, soak them in warm water. Tightly roll, stuff with noodles and vegetables, then serve with hoisin sauce.

Nutritional Information

Calories: 80 per serving
Fat: 1g
Protein: 2g
Carbohydrates: 18g
Fiber: 2g
Cholesterol: 0mg

Roasted Chickpeas

Servings: 4
Cooking Time: 30 minutes
Prep Time: 10 minutes
Total Time: 40 minutes

Ingredients

2 cans (15 oz each) chickpeas, drained and rinsed
2 tablespoons olive oil
1 teaspoon cumin
1 teaspoon paprika
Salt and pepper to taste

Instructions

1. Set oven temperature to 200°C/400°F.
2. After patting the chickpeas dry, combine them with olive oil, salt, pepper, cumin, and paprika.
3. Roast, stirring halfway through, for 30 minutes on a baking sheet.

Nutritional Information

Calories: 180 per serving
Fat: 7g
Protein: 7g
Carbohydrates: 22g
Fiber: 6g
Cholesterol: 0mg

Mixed Berry Smoothie Popsicles

Servings: 6
Cooking Time: 0 minutes
Prep Time: 10 minutes
Total Time: 6 hours (including freezing)

Ingredients

2 cups mixed berries (strawberries, blueberries, raspberries)
1 cup Greek yogurt
2 tablespoons honey
Popsicle molds

Instructions

1. Smoothly blend the berries, Greek yogurt, and honey.
2. Fill popsicle molds, then freeze for a minimum of six hours.

Nutritional Information

Calories: 80 per serving
Fat: 2g
Protein: 3g
Carbohydrates: 14g
Vitamin C: 15mg
Cholesterol: 5mg

Trail Mix

Servings: 8
Cooking Time: 0 minutes
Prep Time: 5 minutes
Total Time: 5 minutes

Ingredients

1 cup almonds
1 cup walnuts
1 cup dried cranberries
1/2 cup dark chocolate chips
1/2 cup pumpkin seeds

Instructions

1. Combine pumpkin seeds, chocolate chips, walnuts, cranberries, and almonds in a bowl.
2. To make a quick and healthful snack, store in an airtight container.

Nutritional Information

Calories: 220 per serving
Fat: 18g
Protein: 6g
Carbohydrates: 15g
Fiber: 3g
Cholesterol: 0mg

Stuffed Mini Bell Peppers

Servings: 4
Cooking Time: 20 minutes
Prep Time: 15 minutes
Total Time: 35 minutes

Ingredients

12 mini bell peppers, halved and seeds removed
1 cup cream cheese, softened
1/2 cup cheddar cheese, shredded
2 green onions, finely chopped
Salt and pepper to taste

Instructions

1. Set oven temperature to 190°C/375°F.
2. Combine cream cheese, cheddar cheese, green onions, pepper, and salt in a bowl.
3. Stuff the mixture into the halves of small bell peppers and bake for 20 minutes.

Nutritional Information

Calories: 180 per serving
Fat: 15g
Protein: 6g
Carbohydrates: 7g
Vitamin C: 100mg
Cholesterol: 40mg

Cucumber Slices with Tzatziki

Servings: 4
Cooking Time: 0 minutes
Prep Time: 10 minutes
Total Time: 10 minutes

Ingredients

2 cucumbers, thinly sliced
1 cup Greek yogurt
1/2 cucumber, finely diced
1 clove garlic, minced
1 tablespoon fresh dill, chopped
Salt and pepper to taste

Instructions

1. To create tzatziki, take a bowl and mix together Greek yogurt, sliced cucumber, chopped garlic, dill, salt, and pepper.
2. Place cucumber slices and tzatziki on a platter.

Nutritional Information

Calories: 60 per serving
Fat: 2g
Protein: 3g
Carbohydrates: 8g
Fiber: 1g
Cholesterol: 5mg

Almond and Dark Chocolate Clusters

Servings: 6
Cooking Time: 10 minutes
Prep Time:** 5 minutes
Total Time: 15 minutes

Ingredients

1 cup almonds
1/2 cup dark chocolate, melted
Sea salt for sprinkling

Instructions

1. Coat almonds in melted dark chocolate by mixing them together.
2. Transfer clusters to a pan lined with parchment paper, top with sea salt, and let to cool.

Nutritional Information

Calories: 180 per serving
Fat: 14g
Protein: 5g
Carbohydrates: 11g
Fiber: 3g
Cholesterol: 0mg

Roasted Red Pepper Hummus Wrap

Servings: 2
Cooking Time: 0 minutes
Prep Time: 10 minutes
Total Time: 10 minutes

Ingredients

1 cup roasted red pepper hummus
4 whole wheat tortillas
2 cups mixed greens
1 cucumber, sliced
Feta cheese for topping

Instructions

1. Top each tortilla with hummus.
2. Add feta cheese, cucumber slices, and mixed greens on top.
3. Fold and present.

Nutritional Information

Calories: 350 per serving
Fat: 16g
Protein: 9g
Carbohydrates: 45g
Fiber: 8g
Cholesterol: 0mg

Tomato Basil Bruschetta

Servings: 4
Cooking Time: 10 minutes
Prep Time: 10 minutes
Total Time: 20 minutes

Ingredients

4 large tomatoes, diced
1/4 cup fresh basil, chopped
2 cloves garlic, minced
2 tablespoons balsamic vinegar
3 tablespoons olive oil
Salt and pepper to taste
Baguette slices for serving

Instructions

1. Put the tomatoes, garlic, basil, olive oil, balsamic vinegar, salt, and pepper in a bowl.
2. Give the mixture ten minutes to marinade.
3. Spoon over pieces of toasted baguette.

Nutritional Information

Calories: 180 per serving
Fat: 14g
Protein: 2g
Carbohydrates: 12g
Fiber: 2g
Cholesterol: 0mg

Avocado and Tomato Salsa

Servings: 4
Cooking Time: 0 minutes
Prep Time: 10 minutes
Total Time: 10 minutes

Ingredients

2 avocados, diced
1 cup cherry tomatoes, halved
1/4 cup red onion, finely chopped
1 jalapeño, seeded and minced
1 lime, juiced
Salt and pepper to taste

Instructions

1. Gently combine chopped avocados, lime juice, salt, pepper, red onion, cherry tomatoes, and jalapeño in a bowl.
2. Accompany right away with tortilla chips.

Nutritional Information

Calories: 150 per serving
Fat: 12g
Protein: 2g
Carbohydrates: 10g
Fiber: 5g
Cholesterol: 0mg

Greek Yogurt Dipped Strawberries

Servings: 4
Cooking Time: 0 minutes
Prep Time: 10 minutes
Total Time: 10 minutes

Ingredients

1 cup Greek yogurt
1 tablespoon honey
1 teaspoon vanilla extract
1 pound strawberries, washed and dried

Instructions

1. Combine Greek yogurt, honey, and vanilla essence in a bowl.
2. To get a uniform coating, dip each strawberry into the yogurt mixture.
3. Before serving, place on a dish lined with paper and refrigerate.

Nutritional Information

Calories: 120 per serving
Fat: 2g
Protein: 6g
Carbohydrates: 22g
Fiber: 3g
Cholesterol: 5mg

Sliced Bell Peppers with Cottage Cheese

Servings: 4
Cooking Time: 0 minutes
Prep Time: 10 minutes
Total Time: 10 minutes

Ingredients

2 bell peppers, thinly sliced
1 cup cottage cheese
1 teaspoon dried oregano
Salt and pepper to taste

Instructions

1. Arrange slices of bell pepper on a platter.
2. Top the pieces with cottage cheese and season with salt, pepper, and oregano.

Nutritional Information

Calories: 90 per serving
Fat: 2g
Protein: 10g
Carbohydrates: 10g
Fiber: 2g
Cholesterol: 10mg

Chapter 7: Desserts for the Noom Diet

Mixed Berry Frozen Yogurt

Servings: 4
Prep Time: 10 minutes
Cooking Time: 0 minutes
Total Time: 4 hours (including freezing)

Ingredients

2 cups mixed berries (strawberries, blueberries, raspberries)
1 1/2 cups Greek yogurt
1/4 cup honey
1 teaspoon vanilla extract

Instructions

Blend together the berries, yogurt, honey, and vanilla in a blender. Process till smooth. To get a creamy texture, pour the mixture into a freezer-safe container and freeze for at least 4 hours, stirring every hour.

Dark Chocolate-Dipped Banana Slices

Servings: 2
Prep Time: 15 minutes
Cooking Time: 5 minutes
Total Time: 20 minutes

Ingredients

2 bananas, sliced
1/2 cup dark chocolate, melted
2 tablespoons chopped nuts (optional)

Instructions

After dipping banana slices in melted chocolate, arrange them on parchment paper and, if like, top with almonds. Allow the chocolate to set in the refrigerator for fifteen minutes.

Baked Apples with Cinnamon

Servings: 4
Prep Time: 15 minutes
Cooking Time: 30 minutes
Total Time: 45 minutes

Ingredients

4 apples, cored and halved
2 tablespoons melted butter
2 tablespoons brown sugar
1 teaspoon cinnamon

Instructions

Turn the oven on to 375°F. Transfer apples to an ovenproof dish. Combine sugar, butter, and cinnamon; pour mixture over apples. Bake until tender, about 30 minutes.

Chia Seed Pudding with Mango

Servings: 2
Prep Time: 5 minutes
Cooking Time: 0 minutes
Total Time: 4 hours (for chilling)

Ingredients

1/4 cup chia seeds
1 cup almond milk
1 tablespoon honey
1/2 teaspoon vanilla extract
1 ripe mango, diced

Instructions

Combine almond milk, vanilla, honey, and chia seeds. Place in the refrigerator for four hours or overnight. Before serving, place chopped mango on top.

Frozen Grapes

Servings: 2
Prep Time: 2 minutes
Cooking Time: 0 minutes
Total Time: 2 hours (for freezing)

Ingredients

2 cups grapes (red or green)

Instructions

Clean and pat grapes dry. For at least two hours, freeze. Savor these revitalizing, all-natural popsicle substitutes.

Coconut and Berry Parfait

Servings: 2
Prep Time: 10 minutes
Cooking Time: 0 minutes
Total Time: 10 minutes

Ingredients

1 cup coconut yogurt
1/2 cup mixed berries (strawberries, blueberries, raspberries)
2 tablespoons granola

Instructions

Arrange granola, berries, and coconut yogurt in a glass. Layers should be repeated. Serve right away.

Pineapple Sorbet

Servings: 4
Prep Time: 10 minutes
Cooking Time: 0 minutes
Total Time: 4 hours (including freezing)

Ingredients

3 cups pineapple chunks (fresh or frozen)
1/4 cup honey
1 tablespoon lime juice

Instructions

Smoothly blend pineapple, honey, and lime juice. Freeze for a minimum of 4 hours, pausing periodically to stir.

Yogurt and Berry Bark

Servings: 6
Prep Time: 15 minutes
Cooking Time: 0 minutes
Total Time: 3 hours (including freezing)

Ingredients

2 cups Greek yogurt
1 cup mixed berries (strawberries, blueberries, raspberries)
2 tablespoons honey

Instructions

Combine honey with yogurt. Place on a tray with liners. Disperse the berries. For three hours, freeze. Before serving, break into pieces.

Mango and Mint Sorbet

Servings: 4
Prep Time: 10 minutes
Cooking Time: 0 minutes
Total Time: 4 hours (including freezing)

Ingredients

2 ripe mangoes, peeled and diced
1/4 cup fresh mint leaves
2 tablespoons agave syrup

Instructions

Mangoes, mint, and agave syrup should all be blended smoothly. For a flaky texture, freeze for at least 4 hours, scraping with a fork every hour.

Almond and Date Energy Bites

Servings: 12
Prep Time: 15 minutes
Cooking Time: 0 minutes
Total Time: 15 minutes

Ingredients

1 cup almonds
1 cup dates, pitted
2 tablespoons cocoa powder
1 teaspoon vanilla extract

Instructions

Mix dates, chocolate powder, vanilla, and almonds until they become sticky. Form into balls. Put in the fridge for fifteen minutes.

Watermelon Popsicles

Servings: 6
Prep Time: 10 minutes
Cooking Time: 0 minutes
Total Time: 4 hours (including freezing)

Ingredients

4 cups watermelon, cubed
1 tablespoon lime juice
1 tablespoon honey

Instructions

Mix honey, lime juice, and watermelon. Fill molds with popsicles. For at least four hours, freeze.

Berry Compote with Greek Yogurt

Servings: 4
Prep Time: 5 minutes
Cooking Time: 10 minutes
Total Time: 15 minutes

Ingredients

2 cups mixed berries (strawberries, blueberries, raspberries)
2 tablespoons honey
1 teaspoon lemon juice

Instructions

Melt the berries with honey and lemon juice by simmering them. Place on top of Greek yogurt.

Kiwi and Banana Ice Cream

Servings: 2
Prep Time: 5 minutes
Cooking Time: 0 minutes
Total Time: 4 hours (including freezing)

Ingredients

2 ripe bananas, sliced and frozen
2 kiwis, peeled and sliced

Instructions

Puree the kiwis and frozen bananas till smooth. For four hours, freeze, stirring occasionally.

Chocolate Avocado Mousse

Servings: 4
Cooking Time: 0 minutes
Prep Time: 10 minutes
Total Time: 10 minutes

Ingredients

2 ripe avocados, peeled and pitted
1/2 cup cocoa powder
1/4 cup maple syrup
1/4 cup almond milk
1 teaspoon vanilla extract
Pinch of salt

Instructions

1. Put avocados, almond milk, vanilla extract, maple syrup, chocolate powder, and a dash of salt in a blender.
2. Blend until creamy and smooth.
3. Before serving, place in the fridge for at least one hour.
4. Serve cold, with the option to add nuts or berries as a garnish.

Nutritional Information (per serving)

Calories: 220
Fat: 15g
Protein: 3g
Carbohydrates: 25g
Fiber: 7g
Sugar: 12g
Cholesterol: 0mg

Cinnamon Baked Pears

Servings: 2
Cooking Time: 30 minutes
Prep Time: 10 minutes
Total Time: 40 minutes

Ingredients

2 ripe pears, halved and cored
1 tablespoon melted butter
1 tablespoon honey
1 teaspoon ground cinnamon
Pinch of nutmeg

Instructions

1. Set oven temperature to 190°C/375°F.
2. Transfer pear halves to an oven proof tray.
3. In a dish, combine melted butter, honey, cinnamon, and nutmeg.
4. Drizzle the pears with the mixture.
5. Bake until soft, about 30 minutes.
6. Garnish with a dollop of vanilla ice cream and serve warm, if desired.

Nutritional Information (per serving)

Calories: 180
Fat: 5g
Protein: 1g
Carbohydrates: 40g
Fiber: 7g
Sugar: 26g
Cholesterol: 10mg

Blueberry Coconut Chia Pudding

Servings: 2
Cooking Time: 0 minutes
Prep Time: 5 minutes
Total Time: 5 hours (including chilling time)

Ingredients

1/2 cup chia seeds
1 1/2 cups coconut milk
1 tablespoon maple syrup
1/2 teaspoon vanilla extract
1/2 cup blueberries (fresh or frozen)

Instructions

1. Combine the coconut milk, vanilla extract, maple syrup, and chia seeds in a bowl.
2. Give it a good stir and wait five minutes.
3. Give it another stir, then chill for a minimum of five hours or overnight.
4. Arrange fresh blueberries on top of the chia pudding before serving.
5. Savor it cold.

Nutritional Information (per serving)

Calories: 280
Fat: 18g
Protein: 6g
Carbohydrates: 28g
Fiber: 16g
Sugar: 7g
Cholesterol: 0mg

Peach Frozen Yogurt Pops

Servings: 6 popsicles
Cooking Time: 0 minutes
Prep Time: 10 minutes
Total Time: 4 hours (including freezing time)

Ingredients

2 cups Greek yogurt
1 cup diced peaches
1/4 cup honey
1 teaspoon lemon juice

Instructions

1. Put Greek yogurt, chopped peaches, honey, and lemon juice in a blender.
2. Process until smooth.
3. Transfer mixture into molds for popsicles.
4. After inserting the popsicle sticks, freeze for a minimum of 4 hours.
5. Before serving, run the molds under warm water to release the popsicles.

Nutritional Information (per serving)

Calories: 120
Fat: 3g
Protein: 6g
Carbohydrates: 18g
Fiber: 1g
Sugar: 16g
Cholesterol: 5mg

Vanilla Pomegranate Parfait

Servings: 2
Cooking Time: 0 minutes
Prep Time: 15 minutes
Total Time: 15 minutes

Ingredients

1 cup vanilla Greek yogurt
1/2 cup granola
1/2 cup pomegranate seeds
2 tablespoons honey
Fresh mint leaves for garnish (optional)

Instructions

1. Arrange granola, pomegranate seeds, and vanilla Greek yogurt in serving glasses.
2. Continue layering until the glass is completely full.
3. Pour honey over the top.
4. If preferred, garnish with fresh mint leaves.
5. Present right away.

Nutritional Information (per serving)

Calories: 280
Fat: 6g
Protein: 12g
Carbohydrates: 48g
Fiber: 5g
Sugar: 28g
Cholesterol: 5mg

Raspberry Almond Butter Bites

Servings: 12
Prep Time: 15 minutes
Cooking Time: 0 minutes
Total Time: 15 minutes

Ingredients

1/2 cup almond butter
1/4 cup honey
1 cup rolled oats
1/2 cup fresh raspberries

Instructions

Incorporate almond butter, honey, oats, and raspberries well. Shape into little balls and chill for fifteen minutes.

Strawberry Shortcake

Servings: 4
Prep Time: 15 minutes
Cooking Time: 15 minutes
Total Time: 30 minutes

Ingredients

1 pound strawberries, sliced
1/4 cup sugar
2 cups whipped cream
4 shortcakes

Instructions

Pour sugar over the strawberries. Let macerate for fifteen minutes. Arrange the whipped cream and strawberries on the shortcakes.

Mango Coconut Chia Seed Popsicles

Servings: 6
Prep Time: 10 minutes
Cooking Time: 0 minutes
Total Time: 4 hours (including freezing)

Ingredients

1 cup mango chunks
1/2 cup coconut milk
2 tablespoons chia seeds

Instructions

Mango and coconut milk should be blended. Add the chia seeds and stir. Fill popsicle molds, then freeze for four hours or longer.

Chapter 8: Meal Planning and Prepping

Weekly Meal Plans

Creating weekly meal planning guarantees that you eat wholesome, balanced meals all throughout the week, which is essential for effective Noom adherence. Take into account these actions to make meal planning easier:

1. **Set Reasonable Objectives**: Match your Noom objectives with your meal planning. Make sure that your meals are tailored to meet your goals, whether they include weight reduction, maintenance, or general well-being.

2. **Variety Is Key**: Serve a range of items from the green, yellow, and red color groupings. This guarantees a wide range of nutrients and adds interest to your meals.

3. **Portion Control**: Use the color-coding system of Noom to determine appropriate serving sizes. To keep a balanced approach, give green foods priority, limit yellow foods, and pay attention to red foods.

4. **Snack Wisely**: To reduce cravings and preserve energy, schedule wholesome snacks in between meals. Choose foods that are high in nutrients, such as fruits, vegetables, or a little amount of nuts.

Batch Cooking for Noom Success

For those who practice Noom, batch cooking is revolutionary since it offers convenience without compromising nutritious content. Here's how to maximize your batch cooking experience:

Select Recipes That Are Noom-Friendly: Choose dishes that follow the Noom philosophy, emphasizing whole, minimally processed foods.

2. **Portion and Freeze**: Once a batch is prepared, divide it into serving portions and freeze. This aids with portion control as well as preserving freshness.

3. **Mix & Match**: Make adaptable ingredients that can be mixed and matched throughout the week, such as quinoa, roasted veggies, or grilled chicken.

4. **Label and Date**: Label every container in your freezer with the contents and the preparation date to help you stay organized. By doing this, you may be sure that you utilize them before they go bad.

Tips for Efficient Meal Preparation

The secret to successfully incorporating Noom into your everyday schedule is effective food preparation. For a seamless and time-saving experience, adhere to these suggestions:

1. **Prepare in Bulk**: Set aside a set time every week to prepare materials in large quantities. Prepare veggies, marinade meats, and ration snacks to make cooking a regular chore easier.

2. **Invest in High-Quality Storage Containers**: Choose containers that are simple to manage, safe to use in the microwave, and freezer. This makes it easy to grab a quick snack or supper that has been prepared in advance.

3. **Establish a Prep Station**: Set aside a section of your kitchen to prepare meals. To cut down on time spent looking for things, keep storage containers, necessary equipment, and supplies close at hand.

4. **Accept Simplicity**: No complicated recipes are needed to use Noom. Concentrate on making tasty, straightforward meals that can be made quickly to relieve tension and encourage a good cooking experience.

You are preparing yourself for long-term success on the Noom diet by developing your weekly meal planning skills, embracing batch cooking, and using effective meal preparation techniques. The resources in this chapter will help you integrate Noom seamlessly and enjoyably into your daily life.

Chapter 9: Staying Motivated on the Noom Diet

Sustaining motivation is crucial for long-term Noom diet success. Take into account these techniques as you set out on your trip to maintain your motivation and dedication to your health objectives.

1. **Establish Realistic Milestones**: Divide your overarching objective into more manageable benchmarks. Honor every accomplishment, whether it is trimming a few pounds or sticking to your diet programs. Acknowledging your progress keeps you motivated.

2. **Visualize Your Success**: Envision the benefits that will result from achieving your health objectives. Visualizing achievement strengthens your resolve to stick with the Noom journey, whether it's more energy, a happier mood, or being able to fit into your favorite clothing.

3. **Create a Support Network**: Invite friends and relatives to join the Noom group or tell them about your Noom experience. Along your health journey, having a support system offers accountability, encouragement, and a feeling of community.

4. **Track Your Progress**: Keep an eye on your food consumption, workout routine, and weight reduction by using Noom's tracking capabilities. Observing observable improvement increases motivation and clarifies the benefits of your work.

5. **Honour Non-Scale Wins**: Honor accomplishments that go beyond the scale. A happier outlook, more energy, or better sleep are examples of accomplishments that enhance your general wellbeing. Honor and commemorate these non-scale accomplishments.

6. **Try New dishes**: Try out some new Noom-friendly dishes to keep your meals interesting. You may avoid diet monotony and increase your passion for eating healthily by experimenting with flavors and ingredients.

7. **Consider Difficulties**: Recognize that obstacles are an inevitable element of every endeavor. Consider the difficulties you've encountered and use them as teaching opportunities rather than obsessing over them. Modify your strategy and proceed with a fresh resolve.

8. **Include Pleasurable Activities**: Mix physical exercise with things you want to do. Making exercise pleasant, whether it be via dance, hiking, or sports participation, encourages you to remain active and improves your general health.

9. **Incorporate Mindfulness Practice**: Make mindfulness a part of your everyday schedule. During meals, be mindful of your body's signals of hunger and fullness, enjoy every mouthful, and be in the moment. A healthy connection with food is fostered and overall pleasure is increased via mindful eating.

10. **Reward Yourself**: Create a system of prizes for reaching certain benchmarks. Give yourself a non-food treat, like a movie night, a spa day, or a new book. Sustained effort is encouraged by positive reinforcement.

Chapter 10: Frequently Asked Questions

Common Noom Diet Queries

Getting around the Noom diet might lead to a lot of questions. To assist you on your trip, the following are responses to some of the most often questions:

1. **Can I follow the Noom diet and still eat my favorite foods?**

Indeed, flexibility is encouraged by the Noom diet. You may still include your favorite meals in moderation while concentrating on nutrient-dense foods.

2. **How does Noom deal with eating disorders?**

Noom uses a behavioral approach to treat emotional eating. Through the program, you may learn coping skills, recognize triggers, and cultivate a positive relationship with food.

3. **Is physical activity a requirement of the Noom program?**

Exercise is not required, although it is recommended for general health. Noom customizes suggestions according to each user's tastes and degree of fitness.

4. **How do color codes in Noom operate?**

Yellow foods are moderate in calories, red meals have more calories, and green foods are rich in nutrients and low in calories. Making balanced dietary selections is made easier by the color scheme.

5. **Can someone with dietary constraints adhere to the Noom diet?**

Absolutely, Noom can accommodate a variety of dietary requirements. The program offers recommendations and support to meet a range of requirements.

Troubleshooting Guide

It is common to have difficulties while following the Noom diet. This is a troubleshooting guide meant to help with typical problems:

1. **Having trouble controlling portion sizes?**

Take a look at Noom's color-coded system and concentrate on mindful eating. To precisely measure servings, use equipment such as food scales and measuring cups.

2. **Experiencing overload while organizing meals:**

Develop your ability to plan meals gradually by starting small. Think about utilizing the program's pre-planned meal alternatives or asking the Noom community for help.

3. **Lack of motivation:**

Review your objectives, acknowledge your successes, and find fresh approaches to maintain your motivation. To make your advancement more attainable, think about changing your milestones.

4. **Weight loss plateaus:**

They are common. Consider your stress levels, workout regimen, and food habits. Breaking through plateaus may be facilitated by making changes in these areas.

5. **Having trouble exercising?**

Find something you like doing, set modest initial objectives, then progressively up the ante. The individualized approach of Noom may assist in customizing workout regimens to your tastes.

Additional Resources for Readers

Try these extra resources to make your Noom experience even better:

1. **The official Noom website**: Keep up with the latest features, advice, and success stories.

2. **Noom Community**: Interact with others, exchange stories, and get encouragement from a group of like-minded people.

3. **Educational Articles**: Noom offers intelligent articles that help readers get a greater grasp of wellness and nutrition on a range of health-related issues.

4. **Noom Coach**: For individualized counsel and assistance, make use of the services provided by your Noom coach.

5. **Suggested Reading**: To enhance your Noom experience, read books and articles on mindfulness, diet, and behavior modification.

Conclusion

Let's review the main advantages of the Noom diet as we come to the end of our investigation into this revolutionary approach to health and wellbeing.

Summary of Noom Diet Advantages:

1. **Behavioral Focus**: Noom stands out for addressing the psychological elements of eating and encouraging long-lasting behavior change with its focus on cognitive restructuring.

2. **Metabolic Enhancement**: By promoting a balanced diet rich in nutrients and individualized exercise regimens, the Noom diet enhances metabolism and promotes slow, sustainable weight reduction.

3. **Color-Coded System**: This creative approach makes it easier to make dietary decisions by directing users toward preparing meals that are colorful, well-balanced, and healthful.

4. **Flexible Approach**: Noom is flexible, enabling users to modify the program to fit their dietary requirements, lives, and tastes.

5. **Supportive Community**: To improve the trip, the Noom community encourages a feeling of connection by offering guidance, support, and shared experiences.

Encouragement for Continued Success:

Recall that change is a process rather than a destination as you go on your Noom adventure. No matter how large or little, acknowledge and celebrate each accomplishment as well as the progress you're making in your life.

Re-evaluating your objectives, seeing yourself succeeding, and using the knowledge you've gained from setbacks can help you stay motivated. Your dedication to the Noom diet is an investment in your health, and its advantages go beyond just weight reduction to include increased vitality, happiness, and general well-being.

Accept the network of support that surrounds you, including your friends, family, and the Noom community. Celebrate your victories, ask for help when you need it, and take pride in the constructive actions you're doing.

Use the resources, tactics, and tools that Noom offers in your quest for ongoing success. These components, which include enlightening articles, individualized coaching, and a lively community, are intended to empower and direct you on your journey to long-lasting health gains.

Recall that the Noom diet is a sustainable way of life that supports overall wellbeing, not simply a band-aid fix. Together with the tenets of Noom, your dedication to making thoughtful decisions sets you up for further success and a happier, healthier life. Best wishes on your Noom-assisted road to long-lasting health!

Printed in Great Britain
by Amazon